29.84

D1631256

Book Supplement to the Journal of
Child Psychology and Psychiatry, No. 1

Editors: L. A. HERSOV and M. BERGER

AGGRESSION AND ANTI-SOCIAL
BEHAVIOUR IN CHILDHOOD
AND ADOLESCENCE

AGGRESSION AND ANTI-SOCIAL BEHAVIOUR IN CHILDHOOD AND ADOLESCENCE

Edited by

L. A. HERSOV
The Maudsley Hospital, London

and

M. BERGER
University of London Institute of Education

Associate Editor

D. SHAFFER
Institute of Psychiatry, London

*Book Supplement to the Journal of
Child Psychology and Psychiatry, No. 1*

PERGAMON PRESS

OXFORD · NEW YORK · TORONTO · SYDNEY · PARIS · FRANKFURT

U.K.	Pergamon Press Ltd., Headington Hill Hall, Oxford OX3 0BW, England
U.S.A.	Pergamon Press Inc., Maxwell House, Fairview Park, Elmsford, New York 10523, U.S.A.
CANADA	Pergamon of Canada Ltd., 75 The East Mall, Toronto, Ontario, Canada
AUSTRALIA	Pergamon Press (Aust.) Pty. Ltd., 19a Boundary Street, Rushcutters Bay, N.S.W. 2011, Australia
FRANCE	Pergamon Press SARL, 24 rue des Ecoles, 75240 Paris, Cedex 05, France
FEDERAL REPUBLIC OF GERMANY	Pergamon Press GmbH, 6242 Kronberg/Taunus, Pferdstrasse 1, Federal Republic of Germany

First edition 1978
Reprinted 1978

British Library Cataloguing in Publication Data

Aggression and antisocial behaviour in childhood and adolescence.
1. Child psychology 2. Adolescent psychology
I. Hersov, Lionel Abraham II. Berger, M
301.43'15   BF723.A/   77-30484
ISBN 0-08-021810-5

In order to make this volume available as economically and as rapidly as possible the authors' typescripts have been reproduced in their original forms. This method unfortunately has its typographical limitations but it is hoped that they in no way distract the reader.

*Printed in Great Britain by
William Clowes & Sons Limited
London, Beccles and Colchester*

CONTENTS

INTRODUCTION TO THE SERIES

L. A. Hersov and M. Berger

The Association for Child Psychology and Psychiatry, a learned society, was founded in 1956 to further the scientific study of all matters concerning the mental health and development of children through the medium of meetings and the establishment of a journal. The Journal of Child Psychology and Psychiatry and Allied Disciplines was first published in 1960 in conjunction with Pergamon Press and this fruitful collaboration has continued over the years.

The Journal is primarily concerned with clinical experimental and developmental studies in child psychology and psychiatry, but its Editors have always recognized the important contributions of other disciplines and other points of view. They have aimed to bring together knowledge from related fields of animal behaviour, anthropology, education, family studies, sociology, physiology and paediatrics in order to promote an eventual integration.

We can claim some success in this endeavour, but have been aware of the need to supplement the material in the Journal with a publication which would bring together, under one cover, research studies on one particular topic or the contributions to a symposium or conference on a particular theme.

In recent years the officers of the Association have considered ways and means of bringing such a publication to the membership and to a wider readership of professional workers in the various disciplines concerned with child health, development, education and care. The Association and Pergamon Press will begin publishing hard-cover supplements to the Journal in 1977. These will appear from time to time under the general Editorship of the Editors of the Journal with the help of an Associate Editor when needed.

The Editors invite contributions of high quality from
clinicians and research workers who wish to publish
their studies in a single volume, as well as the proceedings of conferences and symposia on themes related to child psychology, psychiatry and allied disciplines. All submissions will be assessed through the
normal refereeing process.

Lionel Hersov
Michael Berger

Joint Editors
Journal of Child Psychology and
Psychiatry and Allied Disciplines

INTRODUCTION TO THE VOLUME

D. Shaffer

It is convenient to enquire into aggressive behaviour at at least two levels. Firstly, are there experiences, such as meeting with frustration or witnessing a violent film on television, which will provoke aggressive behaviour in a wide range of individuals? Secondly, are there certain people who are repeatedly more aggressive than others? If so, is this because their threshold for aggressive response is lower than that of others, or is it because they respond aggressively to a different set of stimuli? Is their predisposition to aggression a product of their constitution or their experience?

A good deal of research around these questions has accumulated over the past decade, much of it relevant to the Professional working in a psychiatric clinic, school or other institution. It therefore seemed a useful topic for the 1976 Annual Scientific Meeting of the Child Psychiatry Section of the Royal College of Psychiatrists. The contributions published in this volume are the more complete, annotated, versions of papers presented at that meeting. They have been written by distinguished scientists in a variety of disciplines who report findings of their own research, or make a critical appraisal of the existing literature.

PROVOCATION OF AGGRESSION

Recent research into the provocation of aggressive behaviour has centred on the effects of exposure to televised or filmed violence. Many of the investigations have been with "normal" volunteers, and have often used highly artificial laboratory techniques to elicit aggressive responses. There have been doubts about whether the observed effects are of any clinical importance and, in particular, whether they persist or generalise. There has also been uncertainty about whether the content of the filmed material and, in particular, the extent to which portrayed violence is depicted as justified or unfair, will influence the viewer's response, and whether the response will vary with the viewer's habitual level of aggressiveness. The studies described by Berkowitz in this volume are helpful in clarifying some of

ix

these issues. The subjects studied were not "normals", but
rather Juvenile Delinquents, and the investigations have included both naturalistic and laboratory observations. Account has
been taken of both the content of the filmed material and of the
viewer's habitual levels of aggression, and particular emphasis
has been placed on the persistence and generalisation of effects.

PERSISTENT AGGRESSION

The notion of aggressiveness as an enduring or persisting trait
is one that the two developmental studies in this collection are
especially well equipped to investigate. Manning describes very
detailed behavioural observations among a small group of children
studied repeatedly between the ages of 4 and 7. Farrington draws
data from the Cambridge Study into Delinquent Development, which
has followed a representative sample of boys from 8 until 21
years. Both of these studies show aggressive behaviour persisting across childhood and adolescence, and thus provide empirical
support to the notion of an aggressive character trait. The
longitudinal method also provides information relevant to the
prediction of later problems.

It has long been held that persistent aggression is constitut-
ionally determined. Experimental lesions in laboratory animals
can be shown to induce aggressive behaviour and studies on violent adult prisoners have suggested that they have an excess of
EEG abnormalities. On the other hand, studies into psychiatric disorder in children with frank brain damage or epilepsy
have shown that the nature of their behaviour disorder, i.e.
whether antisocial or neurotic, depends more on family and social
factors than on the nature of locus of their neuropathology.
Harris examines the issue of constitutional factors in a detailed,
critical review of the literature dealing with relationships
between EEG abnormalities and aggression. Her review suggests
that most studies have been marred by serious methodological
problems and is helpful in pointing out pitfalls that could be
avoided in future research.

Studies on selected groups of violent offenders over the past
three decades have suggested that aggression is often associated
with social deprivation and parental coldness or punitiveness.
A problem with these studies has been that they have taken groups
of children, usually identified by particular delinquent acts,
and it has been difficult to be sure that the apparent differences
between aggressive and non-aggressive children were not in some

way artefacts of the selection process. One of the strengths
of the Cambridge study, described by Farrington, has been that
it has studied the appearance of aggressive behaviour in a total
population. The findings published in this volume suggest that
many of the factors shown by aggressive children are similar,
except perhaps in degree, to those shown by children who show
other forms of non-aggressive antisocial behaviour. Most strik-
ingly, the aggressive children had harsh and cold parents, came
from poor, overcrowded and unhappy homes, and did badly at
school. These factors are also the subject of Rutter's paper
which draws upon four important epidemiological studies to examine the independence of and interactions between family, school
and area adversity in determining antisocial disorder. The paper
also lays emphasis on the importance of identifying factors which
allow children to develop normally in the presence of disadvantage.

It is not easy to understand why social, family and school disadvantage should become translated into specific acts of aggressiveness rather than say into unhappiness or withdrawal. Is it
that the child's behaviour is modelled on the aggression of
parents or neighbours? Does the aggression stem from the large
number of frustrations that the disadvantaged child experiences?
Or is aggressive behaviour the child's way of satisfying unmet
needs for attention and respect? Yule, in his review of social
learning research, suggests some of the different pathways
through which aggressive behaviour is learned and rewarded.
These carry important implications for treatment which are described in the remainder of Yule's contribution. Treatment is
also examined in Clarke's critical evaluation of the effects of
different forms of institutional intervention upon aggressive
teenagers. Finally, Storr has written a wide ranging review of
human violence and cruelty, which seeks to integrate both traditional dynamic hypotheses and behavioural or social learning
approaches.

It is clear from these papers that although many questions remain
unanswered, there is an important body of knowledge about this
— at times devastating — form of human behaviour, which is of
the greatest clinical relevance. Hopefully, this collection
will serve to provide some of the scientific framework upon
which informed clinical evaluations and interventions may be
based.

D. Shaffer
Senior Lecturer
Dept. of Child and Adolescent Psychiatry
Institute of Psychiatry, London

SADISM AND PARANOIA. CRUELTY AS COLLECTIVE AND INDIVIDUAL RESPONSE

A. Storr

Whilst aggression is an identifiable part of the behavioural repertoire of many species, including man, cruelty seems peculiar to the human species. It could, I suppose, be argued that a cat playing with a mouse is enjoying the exercise of power; but it is unlikely that the cat either hates the mouse or is capable of entering into the mouse's presumed feelings of terror and help-lessness. Indeed, some authorities would not only deny that predation was cruel in the sense in which we use the word of human behaviour, but would remove it from the category of aggres-sion altogether, confining the use of the latter word to conflict between conspecifics.

Whatever view one takes on this, there can be no doubt that aggression serves a number of different functions and is essen-tial for survival, whilst cruelty is not only a blot upon the human escutcheon, but serves no obvious biological purpose. In-deed, one might argue that cruelty is the opposite of adaptive. Edward O. Wilson (1975) has recently argued that reciprocal al-truism in human, and to some extent in animal, societies is an adaptive device likely to promote the survival of each partici-pant. In other words, kindness to other human beings is likely to pay in terms of survival and reproductive potential; or, as a friend of mine used to put it, "Civility is cheap, but it pays rich dividends." Human cruelty, therefore, is a phenomenon which is not only repulsive, but which requires explanation.

Regrettably, the cruel behaviour of human beings is far too common to be explicable in terms of psychiatric abnormality, or even in terms of special social conditions, important though these are. Cruel behaviour is a potential in normal people. But let us look at some of the factors which appear to make cruelty more likely, and begin by considering one kind of abnor-mal person. In any Western society there are inevitably a few individuals who lack the normal degree of control over immediate impulse. These are the so-called "aggressive psychopaths" who commit violent offences of various kinds, and who may show an almost complete disregard for the feelings of their victims. These are the abnormals whom idealists would like to blame for the whole sum of human cruelty, but who are actually too few in

number to make more than a small contribution towards it. We do
not understand all the reasons for the psychopath's lack of control of violence. As with other psychiatric conditions, the
causes are multiple.

We know some suffer from genetic abnormalities; others show
what appears to be a delayed maturation of the central nervous
system, as evidenced by the persistence, in the electroenceph-
alogram, of rhythms characteristic of childhood. Many psychopaths show a failure of socialization, in that they have never
formed ties of mutual regard with others, and thus live in a
world which they assume to be indifferent or hostile to themselves. The development of conscience, that is, of an internal
regulator of behaviour, appears to depend much more upon the
wish to preserve love than upon the fear of punishment. Since
many psychopaths come from homes in which there has been little
love and a good deal of physical punishment, it is hardly surprising that they have not developed a normal conscience. A
child cannot respond to the withdrawal of something which he has
never had; so that it is understandable that those who have
never felt themselves to be loved or approved of are not affected
by disapproval.

Although many psychopaths show both a lack of control of hostility and also an abnormal amount of hostility towards their fellows, much of the cruelty which they exhibit appears to be
casual rather than deliberate. Thus, they may injure someone
whom they are robbing or sexually assaulting because they do not
identify with their victim or care what he or she feels, which
is obviously a different matter from the deliberate exercise of
cruelty. In Holland, criminologists have experimented with con-
fronting violent criminals with their victims. In some instances
this has brought home to the criminal for the first time that
his victim is a person like himself, with the consequence that
he has wished to make reparation (Roosenburg, 1973).

It is possible that we may be able to understand the psychopath's
lack of control over immediate impulse in physiological terms.
Psychopaths are emotionally isolated, even if not physically so;
and, in other species, isolation appears to produce heightened
reactivity to dangerous stimuli, shown by a faster mobilization
and release of systemic norepinephrine (Vowles, 1970). Human
beings who, for one reason or another, have not learned to mix
with their fellows in early childhood, often show inappropriate
aggressive responses, sometimes overreacting because they per-
ceive threat where non exists, sometimes underreacting because

they have never learned to "stand up for themselves". In rodents,
it has been shown that isolation produces a lower level of tonic
aggressive arousal combined with the heightened reactivity to
dangerous stimuli which I have already mentioned; and it would
be worth investigating whether a similar physiological state of
affairs obtains in human beings who have been isolated.

Since psychopaths constitute a small proportion of human beings,
we cannot explain the human tendency towards cruelty by blaming
it upon them alone, though the study of psychopaths may go some
way towards helping our understanding. The second factor pre-
disposing to cruelty is the human tendency towards obedience.
The experiments of Stanley Milgram (1974) are so well known that
I need hardly refer to them. They are summarized in his recently
published book, Obedience to Authority. To his surprise, around
two-thirds of normal people would deliver that they believed to
be extremely painful, possibly near lethal, electric shocks to a
subject whom they supposed to be engaged in an experiment on
the nature of learning because they were urged to do so by the
experimenter. The excuse that they were only obeying authority
is the one most frequently offered by those arraigned for torture or other forms of institutionalized cruelty, from Eichmann
down. Obedience is clearly adaptive in human society as in many
animal societies. A stable dominance hierarchy promotes peace
within a society, makes possible organized resistance or organized escape if danger threatens, and allows for instant decision-
making by dominant individuals. It is impossible to imagine a
human society functioning at all adequately if we did not have a
built-in tendency to obey. However, obedience involving acts of
cruelty does not explain the cruelty of those who give the orders.

At present, throughout the world, the use of torture appears to
be increasing. There are two main uses. First is the obvious
one of extracting information. Second is its use for the control
of political dissent by creating an atmosphere of terror. It is
an interesting and unexplained paradox that, whilst there is today a general consensus that torture is totally inadmissible, it
is more widely employed than ever before. I do not believe that
the tendency towards obedience entirely explains the compliance
in cruelty of those who carry out cruel orders. It is certainly
a powerful factor in military situations: for instance, in cases
like the Vietnam massacres or the recent execution of mercenaries.
But orders to shoot women and children or one's comrades in arms
are often backed up, in wartime, by the explicit or implicit
threat that refusal might bring about one's own execution. Moreover, it is possible to imagine orders which would be resisted

more strongly than orders to kill or torture. If an officer
ordered that his men should eat faeces for breakfast, it may be
supposed that rather few would obey, even if threatened with
dire penalties.

The third factor conducive to cruelty is distance, whether this
be measured in physical or psychological terms. If human fights
were confined to fisticuffs, there would not only be fewer
deaths, but fewer instances of cruelty. A man who is a few hundred feet above his victims in an aeroplane will drop napalm
upon them without many qualms. He would be less likely to produce a similar effect by pouring petrol over a child and igniting
it if he was close enough to the child to do this. Lorenz (1966)
has argued that human beings possess inhibitory mechanisms against
injuring their own kind which are not well developed and which
are easily overcome because they are not armed by nature with
dangerous weapons like tusks or claws. Natural selection has
not allowed for the invention of weapons which kill at a distance.

By psychological distance I mean the human tendency to treat
other human beings as less than human: the phenomenon of
"pseudo-speciation". Many societies maintain out-groups who are
treated with contempt and often with actual cruelty. In Japan,
for example, the descendants of a pariah caste, known as Burak-
umin, are still discriminated against, both socially and economically, although they are no longer labelled as eta (filth-
abundant), yotsu (four-legged), or hinin (non-human) (Wagatsuma,
1967). In a very interesting paper, de Vos (1966) has distinguished between psychological attitudes to pariah groups and
attitudes to those at the bottom of the hierarchy in any society.
Most of us acquiesce to some extent in the exploitation of the
poor and the unintelligent, and are glad to have them do the
dirty jobs of society; this is instrumental exploitation, just
as torture for the sake of extracting information is instrumental. However, exploitation of pariah castes goes further than
this, and is labelled "expressive" exploitation by de Vos (1966).
By this he means the phenomenon of creating an out-group which
acts as a scapegoat for the tensions within a society, just as
individuals may act as scapegoats for the tensions within a family. Pariah castes not only provide a group of people to whom
even the humblest member of the legitimate society can feel sup-
erior, but are also regarded as disgusting and potentially polluting. A member of such a caste, unlike a member of the lowest
class in a society, cannot rise in the hierarchy because he is
not allowed to intermarry. Harshly authoritarian and insecure

societies have a particular need for scapegoats, just as do
harshly authoritarian and insecure individuals.

Pseudo-speciation plays on the universal human tendency towards
xenophobia, a characteristic found also in other social animals
from geese to monkeys. The more easily human beings are rele-
gated to a subhuman category, or perceived as alien, the easier
it is to treat them with cruelty. The S.S. deliberately degraded
concentration camp prisoners, forcing them to live in filth,
often covered with their own excrement. When the commandant of
Treblinka was asked why such humiliation and cruelty was practised, since the prisoners were going to be killed in any case,
Franz Stangel replied: "To condition those who actually had to
carry out the policies, to make it possible for them to do what
they did" (Des Pres, 1976, p. 61).

The fourth factor which influences people in the direction of
cruelty is the treatment which they themselves experience when
children. Throughout most of the history of Western civiliza-
tion, children have been treated abominably. So much is this
the case that a recent investigation by ten American historians
begins: "The history of childhood is a nightmare from which we
have only recently begin to awaken. The further back in history
one goes, the lower the level of child care, and the more likely
children are to be killed, abandoned, beated, terrorized, and
sexually abused" (De Mause, 1976). Studies of parents who bat-
ter their children show that, as children themselves, those parents had been deprived of basic mothering, at the same time had
excessive demands made upon then, and had been made to feel that
all they did was "erroneous, inadequate and ineffectual"
(Renvoize, 1974, p. 43). Feeling ineffectual leads to demands
for absolute instantaneous obedience, demands which small children seldom, and which babies never, are able to meet. A small
child who will not instantly obey is perceived as a threat because it has the power to increase the parent's sense of inad-
equacy, and therefore invites retaliation. Moreover, deprived
parents, paradoxical as this may seem, make demands on their
children for the affection which, as children, they did not
themselves receive, and react with resentment and violence when
the children do not appear to give it to them. Baby battering
is an interesting example of how basic biological behaviour patterns of protecting and cherishing the immature can be overridden
by personal maladaptation. Helplessness is generally inhibitory
of violence in humans as well as other primates; but once violence has begun to be used against the helpless, helplessness
loses its capacity to inhibit and many actually increase the use

of violence. One of the most distateful features of human
cruelty is   that it persists even when the victim is utterly at
the mercy of his persecutor.

The fact that human beings who have been neglected or ill-
treated in childhood seem themselves more prone to treat others
with cruelty argues that much human cruelty is really revenge.
This is relevant to the dispute which still goes on about the
effects of witnessing violence. Does witnessing violence cause
ordinary people to feel violent themselves, or does it simply
disinhibit those who, consciously or unconsciously, are keeping
violent impulses in check with difficulty? This may be the
wrong question to ask. I shall argue that all human beings are
suffering from some degree of inner resentment derived from in-
fantile experience. On the whole I agree with Herrnstein and
Brown (1974) who, in their recent summary of the literature,
come down in favour of the view that witnessing violence is
disinhibitory of violence rather than provocative of it. I
share the dislike which many psychologists show for a so-called
hydraulic model of the mind; but clinical experience makes it
difficult for me to conceive of any model which does not allow
of resentment being in some way "stored-up". If one allows that
an accumulation of irritations during a working day may be ven-
ted or abreacted by kicking the dog, which is surely a common-
place observation, I see no reason why resentment should not be
stored for much longer, even for a lifetime.

The widespread misuse of the word "sadism" has given rise to
the supposition that human cruelty is partially sexual in origin,
and the ubiquitous response to sado-masochistic literature is
sometimes advanced as evidence that cruelty contains a sexual
element. Elsewhere (Storr, 1972), I have argued at length that
sado-masochism is not what it seems: that, to use the terminol-
ogy employed both by Russell and Russell (1968) and by Maslow
(1960), sado-masochism is "pseudo-sex" rather than sex itself,
using sexual behaviour patterns to establish dominance relationships, as happens in other primates. So many human beings in
Western culture show an interest in sado-masochistic literature
or films that it is not possible to argue that such interests
are abnormal. Yet there are some people who are particularly
plagued by sado-masochistic phantasies and who need such phantasies or rituals in order to become sexually aroused. In my
experience, these people have generally felt themselves to be
particularly uncertain and ineffective both in sexual situations
and in most other aspects of interpersonal relationships; and
their fascination with sado-masochism springs from their need

to establish dominance (or to have the other person establish
dominance) before they can venture upon a sexual relationship.

It seems highly unlikely that torturers are obtaining sexual
satisfaction direct when inflicting pain upon their victims, nor
do I believe that riot police have erections when wielding their
clubs. But the dominance which such people achieve through their
cruelty may certainly facilitate their own belief in their sexual potency. Rattlesnakes wrestle with each other in struggles
for male dominance. The winner of such a contest, it is credibly
reported, immediately goes off and mates, whilst the loser is
unable to do so for some time. The human male needs to feel confidence in order to achieve sexual arousal, and this confidence
may be obtained in all sorts of ways, some of them highly dis-
tasteful. But this is not to say that the exercise of cruelty
is itself sexually exciting. Part of the confusion about sex
and dominance must be laid at the door of Freud. Psychoanalysis
has been so concerned with the pleasure principle, and so ob-
sessed with the notion that pleasure must be sensual, that it
has omitted to consider the pleasure afforded by the exercise of
power. In his early writings, Freud does make some reference to
an "instinct for mastery" (Hendrick, 1943). I have suggested
that, had he pursued the subject, we might have had a book en-
titled Beyond the Power Principle.

It seems probable that those who have been harshly treated as
children are particularly prone to treat other human beings with
cruelty, both because they have a particular need to establish
dominance and because they wish to be revenged. It is also
probable that the casualness and neglect with which infants in
the West have been treated has resulted in there being a large
number of persons who have a rather marked propensity towards
cruelty. Anthropologists are apt to idealize the peoples they
study, but it does seem probable that there are still some
people in the world who are relatively peaceful and kind, and
that this may be related to the way in which they rear their
children. I am thinking particularly of the practice of what
has been called "extero-gestation" in which the infant is kept
in close physical contact with the mother, both by day and by
night, until it is independently mobile. Cultures in which this
happens consider it pathological for infants to cry.

However this may be, there are certainly a large number of people
in our culture who produce evidence of having felt, as infants
or young children, that they were helplessly at the mercy of
adults who were perceived as threatening. We have only to look

at myths and fairy stories to discover many instances of violence
emanating from dragons, giants and other mythological figures
who are immensely powerful compared with human beings and who
may be supposed to reflect something of the infant's experience
of the world.

This brings me to the fifth factor which I consider important
in the genesis of cruelty, which is that of fear. Fear is closely related to pseudo-speciation, and pseudo-speciation is related to myth, since out-groups have projected upon them qualities
which can only be called mythological. I mentioned earlier that
pariah castes are believed to be polluting. This of course makes
them creatures to be feared as well as despised. It is remarkably easy for human beings to be persuaded that other human
beings are malignant, evil and immensely powerful. I am by no
means persuaded of the validity of all that is postulated by
Klein (1950) and her followers, but I am convinced that there
is a paranoid potential in most human beings which is easily
mobilized under certain conditions of stress. The other day I
saw a middle-aged man who was being treated for various phobic
anxieties. The ostensible origin of his symptoms was an experience at the dentist. He was lying prone, and during part of
the dental treatment found it somewhat difficult to breathe.
He therefore attempted to sit up, but the dentist pushed him
down, saying "You're bloody well not getting up." He had previously thought that the dentist was somewhat "trendy" and unpro-
fessional, but at this point the dentist's face appeared quite
different. He changed, as it were, into a malign persecutor,
and the patient lost any sense of being able to resist him. He
actually fainted at this point. The situation had been trans-
formed from one in which the patient was seeking help from a
supposedly benign expert into one in which he was in danger of
death from an evil and powerful enemy. This same patient was
an unusually courageous man who, during the last war, had sur-
vived three air crashes without developing phobic symptoms.

We shall never understand human cruelty until we know more about
paranoid projection, a mechanism of mind which is far from being
confined to the psychotic. Conditions of social stress such as
followed the Black Death in Europe or which led to the collapse
of the Weimar Republic not only throw up pathological leaders,
but mobilize paranoid projection on a large scale. The histor-
ian Norman Cohn has made a particular study of this phenomenon,
which is contained in three books: The Pursuit of the Millennium (1957), Warrant for Genocide (1967) and Europe's Inner
Demons (1975). The history of antisemitism is a case study in

paranoia in which Jews are seen not only as potential dominators
of the world, but also as poisoners, torturers, castrators, and
ritual murderers. Cohn (1967) has demonstrated that the persecution of the Jews has regularly rested upon such beliefs, together with the totally false hypothesis that there was an international Jewish conspiracy dedicated to world domination.
"Exterminatory antisemitism appears where Jews are imagined as
a collective embodiment of evil, a conspiratorial body dedicated
to the task of ruining and then dominating the rest of mankind."
Within the last 30 years, so he reports, travellers in the rem-
oter parts of Spain have been informed that they could not be
Jewish since they had no horns (Cohn, 1967, p. 252). Examination
of the statements of Nazi leaders reveals that they had a megalo-
maniac sense of mission in which they were playing the noble
role of exterminating evil embodied by the Jews. When Irma
Grese was taxed with cruelty she said defiantly: "It was our
duty to exterminate anti-social elements, so that Germany's
future should be assured." As Cohn says: "To hear them on the
subject of themselves, one would think that killing unarmed and
helpless people, including small children, was a very brave and
risky undertaking" (Cohn, 1967, p. 265).

The same paranoid process was at work in the great witch hunt
which took place in Europe during the 15th, 16th and 17th cen-
turies. Witches were supposed to destroy babies, to engage in
cannibalism, to practise incest, to worship the devil, and to
come together in a conspiracy of evil at the so-called sabbats.
It was when this latter belief took hold that the persecution
started in earnest, for the conspiracy was supposed to threaten
both church and state. It is interesting that fantasies of evil
refer to activities which infringe rather basic biological pro-
hibitions: the destruction of babies, incest and cannibalism.

In my belief, man's paranoid potential takes origin from the very
helpless state in which he persists for a long time after birth,
together with the extended period of his total life-span in which
he is under the control of others. Szasz (1974) begins his book
of aphorisms by stating: "Childhood is a prison sentence of
twenty-one years" (p. 1). Whether or not one agrees with him,
I think that the relation between childhood experience and the
propensity to paranoid phantasy deserve further investigation.

REFERENCES

Brown, R. and Herrnstein, R. (1975) Psychology. London, Methuen.

Cohn, N. (1957) The Pursuit of the Millennium. London, Secker
& Warburg.

Cohn, N. (1967) Warrant for Genocide. London, Eyre & Spottis-
woode.

Cohn, N. (1975) Europe's Inner Demons. New York, Basic Books.

De Mause, L. (1976) The History of Childhood. London, Souvenir
Press.

Des Pres, T. (1976) The Survivors. Oxford, O.U.P.

De Vos, G. (1966) Human systems of segregation, in De Reuck, A.
(ed.), Conflict in Society. London, J. & A. Churchill.

Freud, S. (1953) Standard Edition Collected Works, Vol. VII,
Three Essays on Sexuality, p. 159. London, Hogarth Press and
Institute of Psychoanalysis.

Hendrick, I. (1943) Discussion of the instinct to master,
Psychoanal. Quart. 12, 311-329.

Klein, M. (1950) Contributions to Psychoanalysis. London,
Hogarth Press and Institute of Psychoanalysis.

Lorenz, K. (1966) On Aggression. London, Methuen.

Maslow, A.H., Rand, H. and Newman, S. (1960) Some parallels
between sexual and dominance behaviour of infra-human primates and the fantasies of patients in psychotherapy, J. Nerv.
Ment. Dis. 131, 202-212.

Milgram, S. (1974) Obedience to Authority. New York, Harper &
Row.

Renvoize, J. (1974) Children in Danger. London, Routledge &
Kegan Paul.

Roosenburg, A.M. (1973) The interaction between prisoners, vic-
tims and their social network, in Wolstenholme, G.E.W. &
O'Connor, M. (eds.), Medical Care of Prisoners and Detainees.
Ciba Foundation Symposium, North Holland, Elsevier.

Russell, C. and Russell, W.M.S. (1968) Violence, Monkeys and
Man. London, Macmillan.

Storr, A. (1972) Human Destructiveness. London, Chatto, Heinemann, for Sussex University Press.

Szasz, T. (1974) The Second Sin. London, Routledge & Kegan
Paul.

Vowles, D.M. (1970) The Psychology of Aggression. Edinburgh,
Edinburgh University Press.

Wagatsuma, H. (1967) The pariah caste in Japan, in De Reuck, A.
(ed.), Caste and Race. Ciba Foundation Symposium, London,
J. & A. Churchill.

Wilson, E.O. (1975) Sociobiology. Cambridge, Mass., and London,
Harvard University Press.

RELATIONSHIP BETWEEN EEG ABNORMALITY
AND AGGRESSIVE AND ANTI-SOCIAL BEHAVIOUR —
A CRITICAL APPRAISAL

R. Harris

Psychiatrists who are concerned with the problem of diagnosis
and management of deviant behaviour in children have often to
unravel complex clinical and social situations including a possible underlying substrate of an organic brain disorder. This
paper examines in particular the contribution of clinical electroencephalography to the understanding and assessment of aggressive and anti-social behaviour.

There is no doubt that a higher percentage of EEG abnormality
is found in children with behaviour disorders than in normal
children. It is difficult to compare the published results from
one author to another for the criteria of EEG abnormality are
often rather loosely expressed and the findings have not been
commonly compared with recordings from normal children obtained
in similar circumstances. The most precise information on the
EEGs obtained from normal children is given in the monograph
published in 1970 by Eeg-Olofsson. There were 928 normal subjects examined, a "child" group of 743 aged from 1 to 15 years,
and an adolescent group of 185 aged from 16 to 21. The criteria
for normality were strict and the selected subjects were recrui-
ted over a 4-year period from a total of 1300 who presented at
the laboratory as "normal". Routine recordings were carried out
and recording during hyperventilation, photic stimulation and
sleep was possible in 85%. Paroxysmal abnormalities were carefully defined by the author and included spikes, sharp waves and
high amplitude slow waves occurring in focal or diffuse bursts.
Fifteen per cent of the children and 4.9% of the adolescents had
paroxysmal abnormalities at some time during their EEG. The
records were also assessed in relation to the presence of a
slight or moderate excess of slow frequency activity for each
given year of life in relation to mean values. If those whose
EEGs showed paroxysmal or excessive slow wave activity were excluded, there were 68% of children and 77% of adolescents who
had a totally "normal" EEG. Although this information was not
available to earlier workers, it was undoubtedly appreciated
that as in normal adults, round about 10-15% of normal children
would show abnormal wave forms in their EEGs at some time.

In individual EEG assessments the minimum one in ten chance of

13

an EEG abnormality must always be considered in establishing the
relevance of the test result to a particular clinical situation.

In addition to the difficulties of evaluating the EEG results
there has often been a confusing presentation of the clinical
problems. For example, in some papers, such as those by Kennard
(1949), Secunda and Finley (1942), Stevens et al. (1968) and
Stevens and Milstein (1970), various types of behaviour disorder
have been considered together. These authors have included
children with additional evidence of organic brain diseases and
it is therefore impossible to assess the role of the EEG abnormalities reported in relation to the behaviour disorders alone.
In 1974, Carvalhal Ribas and his co-workers studied EEGs from
100 children of from 5 to 16 years of age where the behaviour
disorders were limited to irritability, aggressiveness, impul-
siveness and psychomotor instability. There was a high incidence
of 68% with abnormal EEGs, but the sample included 35 retarded
children, three others with known cerebral damage and nearly
half the children had suffered from various kinds of seizures,
and once again it is difficult to evaluate the EEG abnormality
against the selected group of behaviour disorders. Other workers, including Andermann (1966), Dober (1966), Gerson et al.
(1972), Graffagnino et al. (1968), Hansen (1970) and Small (1968),
have made the distinction between neurologically normal and abnormal children but the behaviour disorders were mixed. This
group of papers showed that the EEG abnormalities have tended
to correlate with evidence of neurological impairment rather
than with the behavioural problems. The publications by Aird
and Yamomoto (1966), and Spilimbergo and Nissen (1971) are comparable in that they excluded children with known epilepsy,
neurological defect or an IQ score in the educationally subnormal group or below, but once again the behavioural problems
varied and there were differing criteria for the EEG assessment.
Most of the papers mentioned report an incidence of about 40 to
50% of EEG abnormality in the disturbed children tested.

The difficulties of such studies have to be appreciated. On
the clinical side, working definitions are not always available,
pure behavioural deviations are not a reality and it is common
experience that neurological impairment in children predisposes
to behaviour disturbance, an aspect which has been discussed by
Pond (1961). From the EEG point of view it is equally difficult
to define normality and, as Eeg-Olofsson has shown (1970), the
percentage of abnormal records in the normal population increased
as the investigation extended from the simple resting EEG through
such provocative procedures as hyperventilation, photic stimul-

ation and sleep, with a variable effect of these activations in differing age groups. For example, sleep tended to evoke paroxysmal activity most readily below the age of 10 years.

An attempt was made at the Maudsley Hospital, jointly with the staff of a Remand Home for girls, to analyse the correlations of the clinical, social and EEG findings in a group of teenage girls on remand, comparing a group of 27 referred for an EEG because of some clinical indication, with a randomly selected sample of 51 girls admitted to the Home over the same period of time. Some preliminary observations are given here by kind agreement with the Staff of the Home, Professor T. Gibbens and Dr. J. Corbett.

There appeared to be little clinically to distinguish any of the girls with abnormal EEGs from the others tested, apart from a tendency to have some slight developmental disorder such as enuresis. However, eight of the nine in the randomly selected group with EEG abnormalities were subject to an "Unruly Order" and thus aggressive or acting out behaviour appeared to correlate more with the EEG abnormalities than other kinds of deviant behaviour.

In practice, there were considerable difficulties in classifying the EEG abnormality and in view of Eeg-Olofsson's (1970) work on normal children, slight degrees of asymmetry or slow wave excess can be accepted or rejected as abnormal on purely subjective grounds. This particular study has been bedevilled by a sizeable group of EEGs assessed as mildly abnormal, making statistical evaluation difficult. Studies of male delinquents have been reported by Loomis (1965) and Kido (1973). No particular EEG correlations were noted in the former paper, but in the latter, anterior theta rhythms and posterior slow waves were found in some persistent offenders of 18-19 years and in those who had committed murder.

An example of a typical work-a-day problem of EEG assessment is given in Fig. 1. The subject, a 13-year-old boy, had made an unprovoked serious physical assault on an adult for which he claimed to have "blacked-out". He was said to have suffered previous black-outs but without associated violence. Posteriorly located, bilateral slow wave abnormalities were seen in his EEG in the waking state but no definite spike discharges appeared during hyperventilation, photic stimulation or sleep. This child had other behavioural problems but no neurological defects.

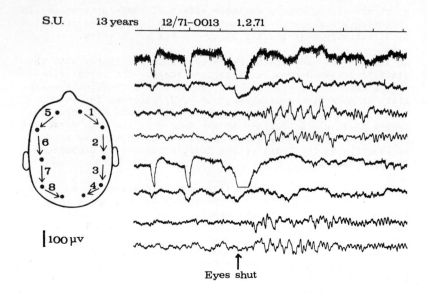

Fig. 1. Bilateral, posteriorly located 3 c/sec
activity seen after eye closure and which did
not show any constant lateralizing features.
This abnormality was present in the waking state
in the EEG of a boy who had made a serious and
unprovoked physical assault on an adult.
(Electrode placement in this, and the other figures, is based on the method described by Pampiglione, 1956.)

Even if it is difficult to understand why EEG abnormalities are
found in neurologically normal but disturbed children it is important to try to assess their relevance in each patient. This
applies particularly to spike discharges for there is a close
relationship with the occurrence of such discharges and clinical
epilepsy, so much so that over the years it has repeatedly been
recommended that disturbed children who have abnormal EEGs without epilepsy should nevertheless be treated with anti-convulsant
drugs. Cutts and Jasper (1939) felt that sometimes the behaviour
disorders were similar to those found in the so-called "epileptic personality". The rationale for drug therapy was also discussed by Gross and Wilson (1964), Itil et al. (1967), Jones et

al. (1955), Lindsley and Henry (1942), and Waller and Kirkpatrick
(1947). Lairy and Harrison (1968) took an opposite point of view.
They followed up 56 of a group of 102 disturbed children who had
spike discharges in their EEG records but no history of clinical
epilepsy. Anti-convulsant drugs were never prescribed and none
of the children developed seizures. It was noted that clinical
improvement, where it occurred, was paralleled by EEG improvement. Unfortunately, the behaviour disorders were once again
of a mixed variety, but the conclusion of course holds for the
aggressive as well as the other disturbed behaviours. Egli and
Graf (1975) followed 76 children over an average period of 9
years who were also disturbed and had spike discharges in their
EEGs but no history of epilepsy. Fifty-six had been treated with
anti-convulsant drugs, 26 for periods of from 3 to 17 years and
none were considered to have improved in their behaviour in relation to the drug therapy. These authors also discussed the disadvantages to these children of being labelled as epileptic and
the problems and dangers of anti-convulsant treatment.

If behaviour disorder combined with EEG abnormality is not necessarily associated with epilepsy, the reverse relationship may
be somewhat different. The interplay of the physiological
effects of epilepsy and the underlying brain damage together
with environmental factors were discussed by Pond (1961). Graham
and Rutter (1968) in an epidemiological survey found an incidence
of behaviour disturbance in 34% of epileptic children with a
significantly greater number of affected children amongst those
who suffered from the psychomotor type of attack. Nuffield
(1961) distinguished various kinds of behaviour disorders in a
group of epileptic children and found that aggressive deviant
behaviours were most likely to be found in those with temporal
lobe epilepsy. The study of 100 children with temporal lobe
epilepsy reported by Ounsted (1969) revealed that 36 suffered
from interictal episodes of rage. The association of aggressive
behaviour and temporal lobe epilepsy is sometimes accepted as a
working hypothesis and it is not uncommon for some disturbed
children who suffer from severe explosive outbursts of aggression to be referred for an EEG in a search for temporal lobe abnormalities even though no overt clinical seizures have been observed. Kligman and Goldberg (1975) reviewed 136 publications
from 1937 to 1973 on the relationship between temporal lobe epilepsy and aggression and concluded that "sample bias, lack of
regard for the validity and reliability of behavioural assessments prevent our deciding whether an association exists between
interictal aggressive behaviour and temporal lobe epilepsy.
Even if this association were demonstrated one could not draw

direct neuro-behavioural inferences from it since a variety of
social and physiological as well as neurophysiological variables
could contribute to the association." Discordance between the
clinical and EEG criteria for the diagnosis of temporal lobe
epilepsy varied from 8% to 34% in the various adult series and
was up to 87% in one of the children's series. Kligman and
Goldberg (1975) felt that the EEG was a relatively crude neurophysiological tool. There is no doubt that the information obtained from the EEG will depend on the extent of the investigation and few authors can compare with the careful pre-operative
procedures in adult patients with temporal lobe epilepsy described by Engel et al. (1975) and which included sleep recording
and various activation procedures combined with sphenoidal elec-
trodes. This type of investigation is perhaps less applicable
to children in whom, as Trojaborg (1968) has shown, spike foci
will change in location over the years in 85%, and in half of
that percentage the change is from one hemisphere to another.

As the association between temporal lobe epilepsy and aggression
is still lacking in definition it may be felt that temporal lobe
EEG abnormalities are also of somewhat tenuous significance in
children. The work of Hill and Watterson (1942), Hill (1944 and
1952) and Williams (1969) demonstrated that in aggressive adult
patients excessive theta activity and EEG evidence of temporal
lobe dysfunction were commonly present, reaching an incidence
of 80% in the habitually aggressive adults described by Williams
(1969). The biological basis of aggression (for which, inci-
dentally, there is no satisfactory definition) is complex and
there is a considerable literature on the contribution of neural
mechanisms which are equally complicated and likely to be modified in each individual by experience and environment. Because
of the prevalence of EEG abnormalities over the temporal lobe,
however, Williams (1969) has suggested that "the prime disorder
of function ... is in the diencephalic and mesencephalic components of the reticular activating or 'limbic' mechanisms, which
have their densest projections to the anterior temporal and
frontal cortex." The experimental evidence for the involvement
of these structures in aggressive behaviour is vast, but unfortunately temporal theta and delta waves, as Driver (1970) and
Eeg-Olofsson (1970) noted, are of such common occurrence in normal healthy children and adolescents that, taken alone, they can
have little value whatever in indicating projected abnormalities
from deep structures or of temporal lobe dysfunction.

Moreover, Stevens and Milstein (1970), in a further review of
100 children with severe psychiatric disorders, confirmed the

Kathleen Th.   17 years   18.3.75   12/75-0120

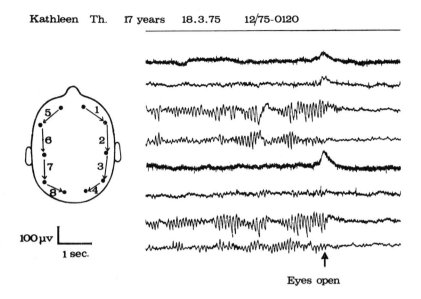

100 μv
1 sec.

Eyes open

Fig. 2.   An example of the commonly seen posterior temporal slow wave focus of adolescence
which is particularly prominent on the right
side. This girl was on remand and complained
of episodes when she was "disassociated" from
her surroundings.

findings of their earlier studies in that they were unable to
demonstrate any association between EEG abnormalities localized
over the temporal lobes with aggressive or anti-social behaviour.
The commonly seen posterior temporal slow wave focus of adolescence may cause difficulties in EEG assessment. Figure 2 is an
example of this wave-form. There are particular considerations
in recording this phenomenon which were described by Wilson and
Lloyd (1973). Using the same normal subjects but differing systems of electrode placement they found that posterior temporal
slow waves are more readily demonstrated with the method described by Pampiglione (1956) than with the internationally recognized 10:20 system. This sort of detail is not often noted in
the literature and yet is clearly important if various waveforms
and their location are to be given clinical significance.

Similar technical considerations are also relevant to the assessment of another waveform, the 14 or 6 per second positive spike
discharge first described by Gibbs and Gibbs (1951) which they
attributed to hypothalamic or thalamic epilepsy. This was said
to correlate with aggression, delinquency and intermittent som-
atic symptoms, such as headaches, abdominal pain and vomiting,
particularly in early adolescence. The EEG techniques for recording these waves are important and require wide inter-electrode
spacing or some kind of average or common reference arrangement
with the subject drowsy or in light sleep as these waveforms
rarely appear in the waking or deep sleep states. Figure 3 is
an example of the 14 per second positive spiking.

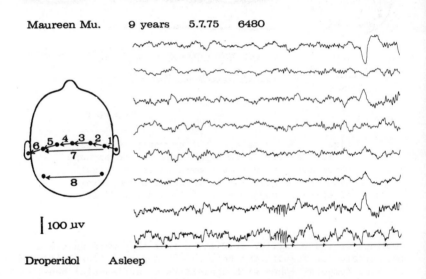

Maureen Mu.   **9 years   5.7.75   6480**

|100 µv

Droperidol   Asleep

Fig. 3. 14 per second positive spikes are
present on channels 7 and 8 (inter-hemisphere
electrode connections). This child was lightly
asleep at the time. She was retarded and
rather withdrawn but had no other behavioural
problems.

A large number of publications supported the Gibbs' hypothesis
and the review by Hughes (1965) reiterated the prominence of

autonomic symptomatology and supported the assumption that the
focus for the discharges was therefore in the thalamic and hypothalamic areas. Henry (1963), however, demonstrated the fallacy
of looking for a common EEG abnormality in groups of clinically
similar patients where the correlations would merely reflect a
particular type of referral. Lombroso et al. (1966) found these
wave forms in 58% of normal 13-15-year-old boys which is a
higher percentage incidence than in most of the reported clinical groups. Eeg-Olofsson (1970), from his wider normal subject
age range, found these waves in 16% of the children and 15% of
the adolescents and in practice these discharges are commonly
found in EEGs in children from about 2 years of age provided the
appropriate recording methods are used. The developmental and
clinical correlates of the 14 and 6 per second spike discharge
were examined in detail in a group of psychiatric patients and
their siblings by Woerner and Klein (1974) without revealing any
meaningful associations. Until more is known about the genesis
of these discharges their ubiquitous appearance means that from
the practical clinical point of view they should be distinguished
from other kinds of spike discharges, but unfortunately in much
of the literature to which reference has been made they are included as evidence of EEG abnormality.

The EEG findings with regard to aggressive and anti-social behaviour in children are therefore less clear than in adults.
The high incidence of EEG abnormality reported in the literature
concerning behaviour disorders generally in children is partly
due to the inclusion of brain damaged or epileptic children.
There is a lack of uniformity in the EEG assessments and no further evidence has been produced which could alter Ellingson's
(1954) conclusion that "no relationships have been established
between EEG abnormalities and specific symptoms". Yet included
in the child and adolescent population are patients who eventually emerge as habitually aggressive adults. A patient of Dr.
Elaine Wright at St. Ebba's Hospital (Surrey), for example, is
now a 20-year-old moderately retarded young woman whose aggression and violence over the years has made her management extremely difficult. Her EEG has always been abnormal. At 12 years
(Fig. 4) there were bilateral bursts of slow wave activity; at
20 (Fig. 5) the slow wave activity was most prominent over the
right temporal regions. She has never suffered from seizures.
Dr. Stern (Queen Mary's Hospital for Children, Surrey) has recently demonstrated that this patient has an extremely rare inborn error of metabolism, gamma glutamide transpeptidase defi-
ciency. It may well be that some consequent abnormality of cerebral function or even damage has increased this patient's vulnerability to disordered behaviour.

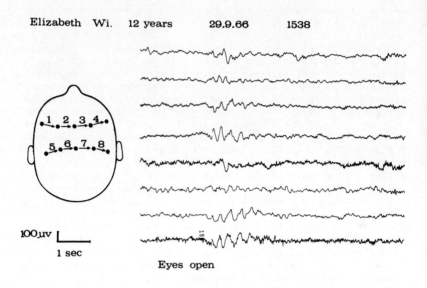

Fig. 4. An example of bilateral 3-4 c/sec
activity in a moderately retarded and extremely aggressive girl who was subsequently
found to have a rare inborn error of metabolism. (See text.)

To evaluate EEG abnormality against a specific behaviour disorder requires a degree of patient selection that has not yet
been attained. Without rigorous investigation, the selection
might well include patients with some undiagnosed organic disease as in the young woman described. Given an ideal patient
group, the EEG findings would need to be set against the odds
for EEG abnormality in a comparable normal population. Until
such information is available, the role of the clinical EEG in
children suffering from disturbed behaviours is still mainly to
draw attention to the possibility of associated organic brain
disorders. However, with the development of EEG services over
recent years, there must now be an accumulation of information
through childhood into maturity which could help in our understanding of the high incidence of EEG abnormalities in habitually aggressive adults.

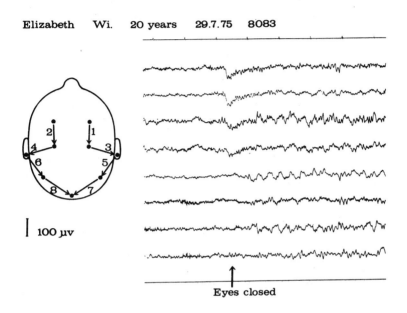

Elizabeth   Wi.   20 years   29.7.75   8083

100 μv

Eyes closed

Fig. 5.   The same patient as in Fig. 4 at 20
years.   During this recording the slow wave
activity was most prominent over the right mid
and posterior temporal regions.   Her extreme
violence had continued.

REFERENCES

Aird, R.B. and Yamomoto, T. (1966)   Behaviour disorders of child-
    hood, Electroenceph. Clin. Neurophysiol., 21, 148-156.

Andermann, K. (1966)   Interpretation of sharp waves and bursts
    of slow waves in the electroencephalograms of mentally dis-
    turbed children, in Wortis, J. (ed.), Recent Advances in
    Biological Psychiatry, Vol. VIII, pp. 257-268.

Carvalhal Ribas, J., Baptistere, E., Vieira Fonseca, C.A.,
    Tiba, I. and Continho Filho, H.S. (1974)   Behaviour disorders
    with predominance of aggressiveness, irritability, impulsive-

ness and instability. Clinico-electroencephalographic study
of 100 cases, Arq Neuoropsiquiatr. 32, 187-194.

Cutts, K.K. and Jasper, H. (1939) Effect of benzedrine sulphate
and phenobarbital on behaviour problem children with abnormal
encephalograms, Arch. Neurol. Psychiat. (Chicago), 41, 1138-
1145.

Dober, B. (1966) EEG findings in childhood behaviour disorders,
Psychiat. Neurol. Med. Psychol. (Leipzig), 18, 405-409.

Driver, M.V. (1970) Electroencephalography and the diagnosis of
temporal lobe disease, in Harding Price, J. (ed.), Modern
Trends in Psychological Medicine, Vol. 2, pp. 326-345.
Butterworths, London.

Eeg-Olofsson, O. (1970) The development of the electroenceph-
alogram in normal children and adolescents from the age of
one through 21 years, Acta Paediat. Scand., Supplement 208.

Egli, M. and Graf, I. (1975) The use of anti-convulsant treatment of behaviourally disturbed children with bioelectric
epilepsy, a follow-up study of 76 cases, Acta Paedopsychiat.
(Basel), 41, 54-69.

Ellingson, R.J. (1954) The incidence of EEG abnormality among
patients with mental disorders of apparently non-organic
origin: A critical review, Amer. J. Psychiat. 111, 263-275.

Engel, J., Driver, M.V. and Falconer, M.A. (1975) Electrophysi-
ological correlates of pathology and surgical results in temporal lobe epilepsy, Brain, 98, 129-156.

Gerson, I.M., Barnes, T.C., Mannino, A., Fanning, J.M. and Burns,
J.J. (1972) EEG of children with various learning problems,
Part 1. Outpatient study, Dis. Nerv. Syst. 33, 170-177.

Gibbs, F.A. and Gibbs, E.L. (1951) Electroencephalographic evidence of thalamic and hypothalamic epilepsy, Neurology (Min-
neap.) 1, 136-144.

Graffagnino, P.N., Boelhouver, C. and Reznikoff, M. (1968) An
organic factor in patients of a child psychiatric clinic,
J. Amer. Acad. Child Psychiat. 7, 618-638.

Graham, P. and Rutter, M. (1968) Organic brain dysfunction and child psychiatric disorders, Brit. Med. J. 3, 695-700.

Gross, M.D. and Wilson, W.C. (1964) Behaviour disorders of children with cerebral dysrhythmias - successful treatment of subconvulsive dysrhythmia with anti-convulsants, Arch. Gen. Psychiat. (Chicago), 11, 610-619.

Hansen, N. (1970) Cerebro-organic pathogenesis in 110 children followed up subsequent to admission to a child psychiatric department, Acta Psychiatr. Scand. 46, 399-412.

Henry, C.E. (1963) Positive spike discharges in the EEG and behaviour abnormality, in Glaser, G.H. (ed.), EEG and Behaviour, pp. 315-344. New York, Basic Books.

Hill, D. (1944) Cerebral dysrhythmia; its significance in aggressive behaviour, Proc. R. Soc. Med. 37, 317-328.

Hill, D. (1952) EEG in episodic psychiatric and psychopathic behaviour: a classification of data, Electroenceph. Clin. Neurophysiol. 4, 419-442.

Hill, D. and Watterson, D. (1942) Electro-encephalographic studies of psychopathic personalities, J. Neurol. Psychiat., Lond. 5, 47-65.

Hughes, J.R. (1965) A review of the positive spike phenomenon, in Wilson, W.P. (ed.), Applications of Electroencephalography in Psychiatry, pp. 54-101. Durham N.C., Duke University Press.

Itil, T.M., Riggo, A.E. and Shapiro, D.M. (1967) Study of behaviour and EEG correlation during treatment of disturbed children, Dis. Nerv. Syst. 28, 731-736.

Jones, E., Bagchi, B K. and Waggoner, R.W. (1955) Focal abnormalities of the encephalogram in juveniles with behaviour disorder, J. Nerv. Ment. Dis. 122, 28-35.

Kennard, M.A. (1949) Significance of abnormal EEGs in disorders of behaviour, Electroenceph. Clin. Neurophysiol. 1, 118-119.

Kido, M. (1973) An EEG study of delinquent adolescents with reference to recidivism and murder, Folia Psychiat. et. Neurol. 27, 77-84.

Kligman, D. and Goldberg, D.A. (1975) Temporal lobe epilepsy and aggression, J. Nerv. Ment. Dis. 160, 324-341.

Lairy, G.C. and Harrison, A. (1968) Functional aspects of EEG
    foci in children, in Kellaway, P. & Petersen, O. (eds.),
    Clinical Electroencephalography in Children, pp. 197-212.
    New York, Grune & Stratton.

Lindsley, D.B. and Henry, C.E. (1942) The effects of drugs on
    behaviour and encephalograms of children with behaviour dis-
    orders, Psychosom. Med. 4, 140-149.

Lombroso, C.T., Schwartz, I.H., Clark, D.M., Muench, H. and
    Barry, J. (1966) Ctenoids in healthy youths, Neurology, 16,
    1152-1158.

Loomis, S.D. (1965) EEG abnormalities as a correlate of beha-
    viour in adolescent male delinquents, Amer. J. Psychiat. 121,
    1003-1006.

Nuffield, E.J.A. (1961) Neurophysiology and behaviour disorders
    in epileptic children, J. Ment. Sci. 107, 438-458.

Ounsted, C. (1969) Aggression and epilepsy: rage in children
    with temporal lobe epilepsy, J. Psychosom. Res. 13, 237-242.

Pampiglione, G. (1956) Some anatomical considerations upon elec-
    trode placement in routine EEG, Proc. Electrophysiol. Technol.
    Ass. 7, 20-30.

Pond, D.A. (1961) Psychiatric aspects of epileptic and brain
    damaged children, Brit. Med. J. ii, 1377-1387 and 1454-1459.

Secunda, L. and Finley, K.H. (1942) Electroencephalographic
    studies in children presenting behaviour disorders, J. Nerv.
    Ment. Dis. 95, 621-625.

Small, J.G. (1968) Epileptiform electroencephalographic abnor-
    malities in mentally ill children, J. Nerv. Ment. Dis. 147,
    341-348.

Spilimbergo, A. and Nissen, G. (1971) Behaviour disorders and
    EEG changes in children, Acta Paedopsychiat. (Basel), 38,
    59-65.

Stevens, J.R. and Milstein, V. (1970) Severe psychiatric dis-
    orders of childhood, electroencephalogram and clinical cor-

relations, <u>Amer. J. Dis. Child.</u> <u>120</u>, 182-192.

Stevens, J.R., Sachdev, K. and Milstein, V. (1968) Behaviour disorders of childhood and the encephalogram, <u>Arch. Neurol.</u> (Chicago), <u>18</u>, 160-177.

Trojaborg, W. (1968) Changes of spike foci in children, in Kellaway, P. & Petersen, I. (eds.), <u>Electroencephalography in Children</u>, pp. 213-225. New York, Grune & Stratton.

Waller, C.F. and Kirkpatrick, B.B. (1947) Dilantin treatment for behaviour problem children with abnormal encephalograms, <u>Amer. J. Psychiat.</u> <u>103</u>, 484-492.

Williams, D. (1969) Neural factors related to habitual aggression, <u>Brain</u>, <u>92</u>, 503-520.

Wilson, S.J. and Lloyd, D.S.L. (1973) The distribution of posterior temporal slow waves: implication of electrode placement systems, <u>Proc. Electrophysiol. Technol. Ass.</u> <u>20</u>, 151-158.

Woerner, M.G. and Klein, D.F. (1974) 14 and 6 per second positive spiking. Developmental and clinical correlates in psychiatric patients and their siblings, <u>J. Nerv. Ment. Dis.</u> <u>159</u>, 356-361.

STYLES OF HOSTILITY AND SOCIAL INTERACTIONS AT NURSERY, AT SCHOOL, AND AT HOME. AN EXTENDED STUDY OF CHILDREN

M. Manning, J. Heron and T. Marshall

This study is an attempt to look at hostility in context, to view it as part of the ongoing behaviour of a child and to consider the role it plays in the life of each individual. This is the approach of the ethologists who have stressed the importance of looking at the whole life-style of an animal before attempting to understand the significance of any one piece of behaviour.

As far as hostility is concerned, there is the complication that this is probably not a unitary piece of behaviour. Among the many definitions that have been proposed, the common feature is that the behaviour is damaging to another person or animal. While we may define damage in various ways, it is perhaps more important to realise that the same damage may have very different "meaning" (in terms of causes, intentions, function) in different contexts. A child may "damage" another by snatching a toy off him. He may do so in a dispute over ownership, he may do so when the teacher has said that all toys must be put away and the victim has not obeyed, he may do so in the role of a restrictive parent in a fantasy game, or he may do so "out of the blue" some time after the victim has annoyed him. If this act is classified in the same way on each of these occasions, then we have lost a great deal of information which might help us to understand the behaviour better.

Because of this it was decided to develop a classification of hostility according to context and to study the children who practised the different types. It was felt that if there were different underlying causes associated with different types of hostility, then those who specialised in one type or another would be distinguishable also in other behaviour characteristics and perhaps too in factors of their home background.

It was also considered important to look at the make-up of a child's hostility as regards the representation of the different types, rather than concentrate on totals. In a given context, children vary in totals because of their varying tendency to initiate or respond to provocation. But they also vary because of differences in sociability (McGrew, 1971; Patterson et al.,

29

1967); an unsociable child lacks opportunity to be hostile and
his total may be low even though he is very hostile on the few
occasions when he does interact.

It is possible that the factors affecting sociability are, at
least to some extent, independent of those affecting hostility
and that the nature of the hostility of the unsociable but hostile child (with low totals) has more in common with a high
scoring sociable but hostile child, than with a low scorer who
is a good mixer, but who only rarely behaves in a hostile way
in spite of much opportunity and provocation.

This project, then, will investigate the proposition that children who have similar proportions of different types of hostility (irrespective of totals), resemble one another in other res-
pects. To allow exploration of many aspects of behaviour, relatively few children have been used. A more comprehensive investigation using larger numbers will follow.

This investigation is in two parts. In the Nursery School Study
a classification is developed; children aged 3 - 5 are grouped
according to their dominant style of hostility and compared for
other behaviour. In the Follow-up Study the same groups of
children are compared at 7½ - 8 years for their behaviour at
primary school and in a family setting. The two studies are
described separately.

I. NURSERY SCHOOL STUDY

(1) Description of Subjects

Fourteen children (nine boys, five girls) were studied at inter-
vals during their second - sixth terms at a nursery school
attached to the Psychology Department of Edinburgh University.
Three extra boys were studied during their fourth - sixth terms
only. They were used mainly in the Follow-up Study but occasionally also in this one.

Three children were from Social Class I and II, six and five
from the two divisions of Social Class III, and three from
Classes IV and V. Two children had no siblings, nine had one,
and seven had two or more. IQ ranged from 94 to 130.

Because of small numbers, this study gives indications only of

the influence of variables of this type. These will not be reported here as they will be investigated more fully in the new
study which is planned.

(2)   Method

(a)   Recording
Each child was observed individually for 1 hour on each of 15
days (three per term for five terms) during periods of free-play.
At such times the children (15-20 in all) played freely with
apparatus laid out in a large hall (sand, water, Wendy house,
boxes, building blocks, paints, etc.) and interference from the
two nursery nurses was minimal. A single observer (M.M.) moved
freely among the children and made two types of record.

1. Diary-type records (two per term, 10 hours per child*) were
continuous accounts, marked off in minutes, of all the child's
activities, particularly social contacts, their initiation,
nature and outcome. The speech of the child was recorded verbatim. This type of record resembles the "Stream of Behaviour"
techniques of Barker (1930) and Barker et al. (1943). It is
relatively inaccurate for fleeting behaviour, but it gives a
good coverage of gross movements and activities. Moreover, it
presents them in sequence which is important for assessing context.

2. Time-sampling records (one per term, 5 hours per child) made
a more accurate check every 10 seconds of certain aspects of the
child's behaviour — those likely to be missed in the Diary records. They were:

Category	Concor-dance	Correl-ation
1. Physical activity: standing, running, etc.	0.92	
2. Social relationship: alone, with one, with group	0.91	
3. Specific activity: type of play, wandering, etc.	0.98	
4. Verbalizations (totals), to whom	0.67	r=0.85
5. Laughing, smiling	0.71	r=0.99
6. Comfort movements	0.62	r=0.93
7. Watching	0.75	r=0.75

* Only 8 hours was obtained for four children.

<u>Observer reliability</u> for the Time-sampling method was calculated
using a coefficient of concordance (Smith and Connolly, 1972).
Product moment correlations for totals are also given for the
more short-lived elements.

It was less easy to assess reliability in the Diary-type method
because two observers following one child closely was distur-
bing. However, this has been done for hostility categorization
(see below).

(b) Classification of hostility

Hostile incidents were recognized and classified directly from
the Diary-type records. First hostility had to be defined. It
was desired to use as broad a definition of "damage" as possible
including, besides physical damage, acts which insulted, inti-
midated, prevented or interfered with legitimate ongoing behaviour.
But because it is difficult for an adult to assess what is damaging in the eyes of a child, an empirical definition was used.
An act was regarded as hostile if it <u>usually</u> evoked a reaction
implying damage. Typical reactions were protest, retaliation,
withdrawal, crying, telling friend or teacher. An act classified in this way was thereafter always treated as hostile whatever the reaction in a particular incident.

Three categories of hostility were established according to context. Their assessment demanded a knowledge of events, especially speech, occurring close in time to the act in question.
The contexts were such as to <u>imply</u> (although they could not
prove) different intent and different immediate cause for the
act concerned. The categories are as follows:

<u>Specific hostility (Sp)</u>: That which occurs in a specific sit-
uation which annoys or frustrates the aggressor. Hostility is
used as a tool enabling the aggressor to get his own way or
assert his opinion. The victim is often incidental. There are
six sub-categories:

  (a) property or territory disputes;
  (b) exclusion of another child from group or game;
  (c) ordering about — a clash of wills over rules or roles;
  (d) precedence — who goes first;
  (e) organization-ordering — insistence on nursery rules;
  (f) judgement — castigation for unfairness, wrong asser-
       tions, cheating or lying.

<u>Harassment (H)</u>: That which appears unprovoked, at least in the
immediate situation and is directed at a person, often the same

person repeatedly. The aggressor may treat the incident as a
joke, even if the victim cries, and he usually attracts the victim's attention to his deed (e.g. a destroyed castle). The
aggressor gains nothing tangible from his act; the "reward"
appears to be the victim's reaction.

    (a)   physical harassment — sudden grappling or gripping (not
           in a game), ruffling hair, throwing sand, etc;

    (b)   teasing — interfering with toys or ongoing activities
           (not because the aggressor requires them), holding the
           seesaw, trampling over sand castle, taunting, jeering;

    (c)   threat — physical or verbal threats of violence or
           hostility   "I'll tell the teacher" or "I won't invite
           you to my birthday party."

Game hostility (G): Rough, intimidating or restrictive activities which occur in a rough and tumble or fantasy game. (The
condition "being in a game" was also strictly defined but details cannot be included here.) Game hostility does not include
normal rough and tumble play, only very rough variants, e.g.
gripping round the throat, hurling to the ground. Also bullying, intimidating or imprisoning against the victim's will in a
fantasy game.

The first two of these categories have something in common with
Feshbach's instrumental and hostile aggression respectively
(Feshbach, 1964, 1970). However, specific hostility, although
"instrumental", is limited to that which is employed to remedy
a frustrating situation "on the spot" and is not the outcome of
frustrations in the past or more generalized aims or grievances.

The third category, game hostility, includes some behaviour not
normally classified as aggressive since play is generally assumed
to be non-aggressive. Without questioning this supposition, it
can be observed that those who overstep the permitted bounds in
a game are strongly resented. Protests such as "You're a bad
boy, you're too rough" or "You don't fight like that" are common.

This classification system as used by M.M. was tested for reliability using the ten separate records of each child in a
split-half reliability test (Spearman Brown prophecy formula);
ru values were as follows:

        specific hostility $ru = 0.945$
        harassment $ru = 0.742$
        game hostility $ru = 0.600$

Correlation coefficients (rho) were also obtained comparing
rank orders obtained for 10 hours' observations with those obtained for shorter periods.

		Specific hostility	Harassment	Games hostility
(a)	3 hours	0.88 $p < 0.001$	0.537 $p < 0.05$	0.953 $p < 0.001$
(b)	4 hours	0.898 $p < 0.001$	0.755 $p < 0.01$	0.825 $p < 0.001$
(c)	5 hours	0.879 $p < 0.001$	0.762 $p < 0.01$	0.957 $p < 0.001$

This suggests that records of less than 4 hours' duration are
not so reliable.

Parallel observations scoring and subsequently classifying hostile incidents yielded concordance coefficients of 0.87 for number of incidents and 0.83 for classification.

TABLE 1
Significant Differences in Totals and Proportions of the Three
Types of Hostility Scored by Each Child in Its First and Second
Year in Nursery respectively
(5 hours per child per year, except for ⌀ children = 4 hours)
Significant differences are indicated by the following conven-
tion: * $p < 0.05$; ** $p < 0.025$; *** $p < 0.01$; **** $p < 0.001$.
All are based on chi^2 calculations. Totals for the two years
were tested against the null hypothesis that they were equal.
Sp = Specific hostility; H = Harassment; G = Game hostility.

Child	Total Sp	Total H	Total G	%Sp	%H	%G	%Sp/Sp+H
Adam	***		****		****	****	
⌀ Jacob							
⌀ Jack	****	***	****		*		
Colin			****		***	***	
Ben			****			****	
Mark		***	****		***	****	
⌀ Luke			****	****		****	
Simon			****		****	****	
⌀ Hilda	***		****		****	***	
Jill							
Alice	****						
Ann							
Derek		****	****	****	*	*	***
Lucy	*		****	*		****	

(c) Hostility groups

The intention to consider proportions, not totals, of the different kinds of hostility was discussed in the introduction. It was necessary, however, to assess the stability of such a measure, particularly over time, since a measure which can only be applied at a certain stage of nursery life is impracticable. Accordingly, the 14 children were compared for totals and proportions of hostility taken from diary-type records 1-5 and 6-10 respectively (when the children were 3-4 and 4-5 years of age). Table 1 shows that both totals and proportions change considerably with time. However, it seemed likely that the main cause of variation in proportions was due to the relatively unstable Games hostility. This, unlike the other two hostility types, is situation limited and the likelihood of being "in a game" varies with age and also, to some extent, by chance. It seemed legitimate to ignore games situations and look at the relationship between specific hostility and harassment in a non-game context. This is expressed as the proportion of Specific hostility in the total of both (%Sp/Sp+H). Table 1 shows this measure to be remarkably stable, only one child changing its value significantly between his first and second year. Hence, in spite of considerable changes in totals, each child tends to maintain a steady relationship between these two types of hostility throughout his nursery career.

Accordingly, this measure was used as a basis for the establishment of the hostility groups. Table 2 shows the children ranked on a Sp/Sp+H scale. This represents a gradual transition from those who are specific specialists at the top to harassment specialists at the bottom, and four groups have been distinguished by arbitrary divisions on this scale. However, it is apparent that the three boys at the bottom end of the scale are remarkable for their high proportions of game hostility. In case this should be significant these were separated from other harassment specialists and called games specialists.

The four hostility groups are therefore as follows:

Group 1 - Games specialists
Sp/Sp+H < 35% Sp < H < G   3♂♂

Group 2 - Harassment specialists
35% < Sp/Sp+H < 50% H > Sp > G   or   H > G > Sp   5♂♂

Group 3 - Teaser-specifics   3♀♀
50% < Sp/Sp+H < 59% Sp equal to or slightly higher than H (+1♂)

Group 4 - Specific specialists
Sp/Sp+H > 58% Sp much greater than H   2♀♀
                                                             1♂(+2♂♂)

TABLE 2
Children Ranked for Sp/Sp+H% Scores and Divided into
Hostility Groups

Child	%Sp/Sp+H	Specific hostility Total	%	Harassment Total	%	Game hostility Total	%	Total hostility
Group 4 Specific specialists = Specifics								
♀ Lucy	69%	82	59%	36	26%	21	15%	139
♂ Derek	63%	39	34%	25	22%	50	44%	114
♀ Ann	59%	13	48%	9	39%	5	19%	27
Group 3 Teaser specifics								
♀ Alice	58%	89	49%	65	36%	28	15%	182
♀ Jill	52%	46	49%	40	43%	7	8%	93
∅ ♀ Hilda	51%	65	45%	64	44%	17	11%	146
Group 2 Harassment specialists = Teasers								
♂ Simon	43%	93	28%	124	38%	110	34%	327
∅ ♂ Luke	42%	49	28%	67	38%	60	34%	176
♂ Mark	42%	82	34%	114	48%	44	18%	240
♂ Ben	39%	54	34%	86	54%	18	12%	158
♂ Colin	36%	27	28%	49	51%	20	21%	96
Group 1 Games specialists = Games group								
∅ ♂ Jack	32%	29	15%	61	31%	104	54%	194
∅ ♂ Jacob	31%	27	18%	60	40%	62	42%	149
♂ Adam	29%	31	14%	75	31%	122	54%	228
Figures for extra three boys used mainly in Follow-up Studies, 5 hours of records only								
♂ Bruce (Group 4) 79%		92	48%	25	13%	73	28%	190
♂ Peter (Group 4) 61%		36	33%	23	21%	49	46%	108
♂ Paul (Group 3) 51%		43	25%	42	25%	85	50%	170

Figures taken from 10 hours of records apart from children
marked ∅ (8 hours).

These divisions are arbitrary and the groups are thus essentially artificial. Nevertheless, it is likely that if the make-up of a child's hostility does have significance in terms of causation, then comparisons between such groups will reveal it.

(d) Behaviour characteristics and hostility groups

The behaviour characteristics which were used to assess differences between the groups were taken from both types of record. Many comparisons were made but only those which show significant differences between the groups are reported here. The characteristics will be defined here and discussed further with the results.

1. Total hostility = all types of hostility.
2. Hostility (non game) = Specific hostility and Harassment only.
3. Total violence = all incidents of hits, kicks, punches or very rough physical handling.
4. Total verbalizations come from verbatim diary records. A single verbalization was categorized as a single utterance (whether sentence or not) of a given functional type (see below). In long utterances, each sentence was counted as a verbalization. Utterances which could not be understood (10-15%) were counted in totals but not classified. The classification is based on that used by Piaget (1926), but it includes more categories. The categories are largely functional, e.g. suggestion, invitation, order, challenge, protest, comment, criticism, etc.
5. Hostile speech = that used in hostile incidents.
6. Friendly speech = categories such as greeting, invitation, comment, suggestion.
7. Objective speech (Ob. speech) is about objective matters, books, pictures, TV programmes, events, etc.
8. Self-oriented speech (S. speech) is concerned with the child's own activities (excluding monologues), past, present and future.
9. Interactive speech (Int. speech) is concerned with relationships between children of all types (ordering, persuading, agreeing, arguing, insulting, etc.).
10/11. Suggestions, Invitations and Orders are shown here as totals for the second year only (using 17 children) because the totals for the 14 children did not discriminate the groups. In this analysis group 2 (Harassment specialists) are divided into sections (a) H > Sp > G and (b) H > G > Sp.
12. % success in disputes. A dispute situation is one in which

there is a clash of interests. This is a measure of the
proportion of such disputes involving one child which he
won. Disputes with ambiguous outcomes were ignored.

In this study the children have been ranked for their totals of
these various behaviour characteristics. Usually the totals are
for 10 hours (5 hours if for year 2). The totals of the four
children for whom there are only 8 hours of records have been
adjusted proportionally. It is then considered whether or not
members of a given hostility group appear at random on this rank
scale or if they cluster at the top or bottom. Significant differences between hostility groups have been computed using the
Mann-Whitney U test (one-tailed).

(3)   Results and Discussion

Table 3 shows the results of these comparisons. For each behaviour characteristic the scores of individual children are given
in rank order (from left to right). The children are not named
(for lack of space), but the hostility group and sex (if ♀) of
the child is indicated below each score. To the right, significant differences between the hostility groups are given. Wherever two hostility groups can be distinguished from the remaining two, the probability of this is written in full. If, in
addition, one group ranks significantly higher or lower than the
rest, it is marked by *s with the following meaning: * $p < 0.05$;
** $p < 0.025$;   *** $p < 0.01$;   **** $p < 0.001$.

Thus,   *4+1>2+3***
                          $p < 0.001$

means groups 4+1>2+3 $p < 0.001$;   4>1+2+3 $p < 0.05$;   3<1+2+4 $p < 0.01$.

Sex differences are also given where they are significant. In
this sample, groups 1 and 2 are all male and groups 3 and 4 mainly female. Hence it is necessary to consider the possibility
that behavioural differences between these groups may be related
to sex rather than hostility differences. Some comments should
be made about the comparisons.

(1, 2, 3). Boys score significantly higher than girls in total
hostility although not in violence. However, boys play more
rough games than girls; and some score highly in games hostility. In non-game contexts, the sex difference disappears. It
is also apparent that the high hostility of the Games group
occurs mainly in games situations while that of the Teasers
occurs at all times.

TABLE 3

Rank Orders of Scores for Various Behaviour Characteristics
Labelled According to the Hostility Group and Sex of the Child
(for explanation see text, p. 38)

♀♀ are marked.
Hostility groups numbers are written below the score:
Gp 1 = Games group;   Gp 2 = Teasers;
Gp 3 = Teaser-specifics;   Gp 4 = Specifics.

Characteristic	Scores	Significance
. Total host. 10 hrs	327-242-240-228-220-186-183-182-158-139-114- 96- 93- 27 2 - 1 - 2 - 1 - 2 - 1 - 3♀- 3♀- 2 - 4♀- 4 - 2 - 3♀- 4♀	♂ > ♀ * 1+2>3+4* p < 0.01
. Host. (non-game)	217-196-154-161-145-140-118-112-109-106- 86- 76- 64- 22 2 - 2 - 3♀- 3♀- 2 - 2 - 4♀- 1 - 1 - 1 - 3♀- 2 - 4 - 4♀	2+3>1+4* p < 0.025
. Total violence 10 hrs	22- 16- 14- 13- 13- 7- 7- 4- 3- 2- 2- 1- 0- 0 2 - 1 - 3♀- 1 - 2 - 1 - 2 - 2 - 2 - 4♀- 3♀- 3♀- 4 - 4♀	1+2>3+4** p < 0.01
a. Total verb. 10 hrs	1383-1158-917-902-870-845-751-702-689-619-615-603-456-432 4♀- 3♀- 4♀- 2 - 3♀- 2 - 4 - 1 - 2 - 3♀- 1 - 1 - 2 - 2	*4+3>2+1 p < 0.025 ♀ > ♂ **
b. Total verb. Year 2 with extra boys, 5 hrs	813-725-592-538-521-514-481-471-468-425-400-393-360-323-265-260-260 4♀- 3♀- 4 - 2 - 4♀- 4 - 4 - 2 - 3♀- 2 - 1 - 3♀- 1 - 3 - 1 - 2 - 2	***4+3>2+1 p < 0.025
. Total hostile speech, 10 hrs	139-127-123-116-111-110- 72- 63- 62- 58- 49- 47- 40- 18 3♀- 3♀- 4♀- 2 - 3♀- 2 - 1 - 2 - 1 - 2 - 1 - 2 - 4 - 4♀	3 > rest**
. Total friendly speech, 10 hrs	915-709-552-534-519-445-413-340-311-256-238-235-222-198 4♀- 3♀- 2 - 4♀- 1 - 4 - 2 - 3♀- 2 - 1 - 2 - 1 - 3♀- 2	4 > rest*
. Total ob. speech, 10 hrs	198-194-149-140-113- 98- 95- 69- 62- 60- 48- 47- 41- 35 4♀- 1 - 4♀- 2 - 3♀- 4 - 3♀- 2 - 2 - 1 - 2 - 1 - 3♀- 2	4 > rest*
. Total s. speech 10 hrs	320-187-181-129-127- 99- 96- 89- 79- 77- 71- 70- 64- 34 4♀- 4♀- 3♀- 4 - 3♀- 2 - 2 - 1 - 1 - 1 - 2 - 2 - 2 - 3♀	***4+3>1+2 p < 0.025
a. Total int. speech, 10 hrs	577-540-495-327-299-297-285-275-249-245-233-225-177-149 4♀- 3♀- 2 - 2 - 2 - 3♀- 1 - 1 - 4 - 1 - 3♀- 4♀- 2 - 2	no sig. diffs.
b. % int. speech	76- 70- 68- 68- 65- 65- 65- 64- 57- 56- 53- 52- 50- 40 3♀- 2 - 1 - 2 - 1 - 3♀- 2 - 2 - 3♀- 2 - 4♀- 4 - 1 - 4♀	1+2+3>4** p < 0.025
0. Sugg. + inv. in 5 hrs. Year 2 with extra boys	43- 36- 31- 30- 26- 26- 24- 23- 17- 16- 15- 13- 11- 10- 9- 9- 2 3♀- 4♀- 4 - 2b- 2a- 2b- 4 - 4♀- 4 - 1 - 3♀- 3 - 1 - 2a- 1- 3♀- 2a	4+2b > rest p < 0.01 4+2 > rest p < 0.025 F
1. Sugg. inv. orders 5 hrs. Year 2 with extra boys	154-106-102- 63- 61- 58- 57- 55- 55- 50- 45- 43- 35- 33- 31- 24- 18 4 - 4♀- 3♀- 2b- 2b- 1 - 3♀- 4♀- 4 - 2a- 4 - 1 - 3 - 1 - 3♀- 2a- 2a	4+2b+3 > rest p < 0.025
2. % success in disputes	77- 77- 68- 64- 59- 58- 57- 57- 54- 50- 45- 43- 40- 34 2 - 3♀- 2 - 2 - 2 - 4♀- 4♀- 4 - 3♀- 1 - 2 - 1 - 1 - 3♀	*2+4>3+1* p < 0.05

Significant differences based on Mann-Whitney U Test (one-tailed)
unless marked F (= Fisher Exact Probability test).

(4a,b). Among the 14 children, girls talk more than boys (4a).
But this sex difference disappears when 17 children are used
(year 2 — 4b), while the ascendancy of the Specifics is confirmed. Apparently boy Specifics, as well as girls, talk a lot.

(5). The hostility of all the girls in this study is proportionally more verbal (and less physical) than that of the boys
(p < 0.001). However, it is the Teaser-specifics who have the
highest totals of hostile speech.

(6, 7, 8). Specifics stand out in all these aspects of affil-
iative speech. Objective and self-oriented speech may well make
their speech more interesting. These children are often doing
things (painting, building) and talk about their activities.

(9a,b). Totals of interactive speech do not distinguish the
groups but the Specifics have proportionally less than others.
Where there are high proportions (65%+), children seem too concerned with social relationships to talk of much else. This
study shows them to be also inept, largely unfriendly and unsuccessful. Specifics are relatively less concerned and more successful.

(10, 11). These are measures of persuasiveness (10) or more
dominating "bossiness" (11). Teaser-specifics feature in the
latter but not in the former. High scorers in (10) could become popular leaders (Kummer, 1968; Saayman, 1971; Slater,
1955; Davis, 1961), and some Specifics have been seen to organize the whole nursery into a single game. The less withdrawn
of the Teasers (2b) could also be persuasive but they were
usually too unpopular to become leaders.

(12). This gives some measure of dominance as in traditional
hierarchies (Carpenter, 1965; Hall and deVore, 1965, Goodall,
1968). High scorers tend to be high in Sp and H but not G. It
is not surprising that the Teasers head the rank order; the
Games group by contrast are remarkably unsuccessful.

These findings, although based on relatively few behaviour
characteristics and applied to a small sample of children, are
nevertheless sufficiently consistent among themselves to provide
a coherent picture of the characteristics of the different hostility groups.

Group 1 = Games specialists show high totals of hostility and
violence but these are scored mainly in the game situation. In

games these children tend to become wild and "out of control". Outside of a game they are observably timid, talk relatively little (4a,b), make few attempts to organize others (10, 11) and are unsuccessful in disputes (12).

Group 2 = Harassment specialists = Teasers are among the most hostile and violent children in the nursery (1, 2, 3). They talk relatively little and their speech is low in the more interesting objective and self-oriented remarks (4a,b, 7, 8). They are dominating and successful in disputes (12). Some of them are persuasive (10) but none (in this study) became a leader.

Group 3 = Teaser-specifics tend to be bossy as well as teasing. Their high hostility is mainly outside the game situation and they are not violent (2, 3). But they tend to be hostile in their speech (5) and to organize in a dominating rather than a persuasive way (11). They talk a lot (4a,b) and quite a lot about themselves (8) but they are not so high in objective speech (9). They are also relatively unsuccessful in disputes (12).

Group 4 = Specific specialists appear to be the best adapted children socially. Most of them show relatively low hostility and little violence in all situations (1, 2, 3). They talk a lot and much of their speech is friendly and interesting (4a,b, 5, 6, 7, 8). When they organize, some are bossy but most can be persuasive too and some become leaders of the class (10, 11). As a group these children seem least concerned about their relationships with others, as indicated by their speech (9b).

It is arguable that, with the small numbers of children in each group, many of the correlations demonstrated above could be due to chance. It is unlikely, however, that so many should appear which are so consistent with one another, even allowing for the fact that certain of the characteristics have qualities in common. To test this the children were assigned to four random groups A, B, C, D (by pulling their names out of a hat) although it was arranged that the new groups resembled the hostility groups in sex composition. 4/14 of the Behaviour Characteristics listed in Table 3 showed significant differences for A, B, C, D (13/14 for hostility groups). These yielded no coherent picture other than the fact that As were more aggressive.

II. FOLLOW-UP STUDIES

(1) Introduction

The nursery study suggests that children who have different
styles of hostility also differ in other aspects of their social
behaviour. Only the specific specialists seem socially well-
adjusted. Specific hostility seems to resemble Kelly's aggressive behaviour which he describes as an "outgoing exploratory
activity" (Kelly, 1970). It is functional in that it seems to
help an assertive child manipulate his environment (within limits) and as such it resembles the aggressive behaviour of most
animals which Lorenz has shown to be biologically adaptive
(Lorenz, 1966; Johnson, 1972). By contrast, the "aim" of
harassment seems to be the discomfiture of the victim. While
it is often successful in this, the goal does not seem to be a
biologically adaptive one. Teasers are unpopular and are social
misfits. The game specialists would seem to have a similar "aim"
but it is coupled with a strong desire to please, hence their
hostility is disguised in a game.

In short, it is suggested that all types of hostility, other
than specific hostility, is to some extent maladaptive and may
have its roots in distorted social relations at home. Every
child shows some instances of these maladaptive types, but when
they are dominant, there may be cause for concern. In so far
as disturbed social factors may be continuing, it is likely that
both the aggression and the associated behaviour will also persist. The follow-up study was designed to test all these implications. It aimed to look at the child's social behaviour at
home and at school at the age of 7-8 years, to test for signs
of disturbed behaviour in both these settings and to enquire
into the nature of the home environment.

(2) Subjects

All 17 children were included in this study (the original 14
together with the three extra boys). This made the group composition as follows:

> Group 1 = Games group: three boys
> Group 2 = Teasers: five boys
> Group 3 = Teaser specifics: one boy, three girls
> Group 4 = Specifics: three boys, two girls

The children were studied when between the ages of 7 and 8, mostly at about 7½ years.

(3) Method

The following investigations were made:

A. School Studies (with Mrs Thompson, Mrs Barlow, Mrs Gower)

a. **Playground observations** — for comparison with nursery studies. Two hours of observation were made by M.M. on each child separately during unsupervised playtime. The children could not be hostility-typed as it was not possible to hear what was said. Instead social behaviour was assessed using a time-sampling technique. This will be reported more fully elsewhere.

b. **Rutter questionnaire for teachers** (Rutter, 1967) — to assess disturbed behaviour at school. Questions were asked on 26 behaviour traits (of 7 - 13-year-olds) and the teacher had to make ratings: certainly applies (2 points); applies somewhat (1 point); or doesn't apply (0 points). Rutter found that about half the children who scored over 9 points in his study had definite psychiatric disorders, while this was true of only 2.3% of those scoring below 9.

c. **Teacher structured questions** — to assess more positive aspects of the child's behaviour. Questions were asked on co-operativeness, self-confidence, ability, emotionality, appearance, etc., and teachers were again required to reply on a three-point scale. Individual questions were grouped to measure wider characteristics.

Enquiries b and c were conducted by three assistants, none of whom had any prior knowledge of the children. Two (in one case three) teachers were approached for each child to minimize teacher bias.

B. Home Enquiries (with Judi Heron, Tina Marshall, Pat Thompson)

a. **The behaviour inventory** (Wolff, 1967) — to assess disturbed behaviour at home. Dr Judi Heron, a psychiatrist, conducted a structured interview with each mother enquiring about 25 behaviour characteristics of her child. They were scored on a five-point scale, previously tested for reliability by Dr Wolff, who had also shown that for all these traits, disturbed children (referred to a psychiatric clinic) scored significantly higher than normals (p < 0.01). In this study, replies were written down and scored independently by Judi Heron (J.H.), Tina Marshall (T.M.) and Margaret Manning (M.M.) (only M.M. knew the children). Agreement was as follows:

between M.M. and J.H.   80%
        M.M. and T.M.   76%
        J.H. and T.M.   75%

Number of items within one point of difference 372/395 = 95%.

b. The standard day interview — to assess typical home interactions. This was a modification of Douglas's technique (Douglas et al. 1968a,b) which was designed for use with younger children. Tina Marshall interviewed each mother on two occasions and took her through the events of the previous evening (after school). The interview was recorded and data was used to measure amounts and intensities of family interactions (using Douglas's classification) and totals of certain activities — conversations, arguments, fights, nurturant activities, play, etc. The reliability of such counts depends upon the ability and willingness of the mother to report them. They were used mainly as supportive evidence.

c. Mother structured questions — to enquire about mothers' attitudes and about environmental and birth history. Tina Marshall and Judi Heron conducted two separate enquiries here. The first, which was recorded, consisted of open-ended questions about conflicts in the home, interests in common with the child, his outside activities and friends. This data was also used as supportive evidence. Judi Heron employed a standard set of questions used by psychiatrists.

d. Family structured interview = Tea-party — to provide opportunity for direct observation of family interactions. The mother and all her children were invited to a tea-party where the mother was first asked to get her children to play four games which were set out. She could join in or not as she wished and the session (lasting 30 minutes) was video-taped through a one-way screen. One observer stayed with the family.

Sixteen children were observed (Bruce (Specific) was not available). Two separate tea-parties were held for the two siblings in the study, Jack and Jill. Peter and Mark, without siblings, invited friends (their results were omitted from intersibling comparisons). There are many facets to

the analysis. Here only three will be described. They are
(1) speech analysis, (2) mother's controlling behaviour,
(3) evidence of favouritism.

(1) Speech analysis. Speech (from the video-tape records)
was analysed into functional categories as in the nursery
study. They were grouped into the following larger classes:
positive speech; negative speech; nurturant speech; organizing speech; competitive speech; conversation (= all
positive speech except organizing, praise and judgement).
Tone of voice was assessed as positive, negative, attention-
seeking or neutral by agreement between M.M. and T.M. No
objective significance can be claimed here, but the results
are included for interest. The children and mothers were
compared for the nature of their speech to different members
of the family. Very large differences in speech totals were
found which were reflected in every rank order of speech
categories. Consideration of the proportional (%) representation of the different categories, however, gave a picture
of the flavour of speech, i.e. whether it was more or less
nurturant or negative, irrespective of totals. This measure
was often used.

(2) Controlling methods used by the mother were considered
under four headings:

Manipulation = manhandling of child or its toy.
Physical control = wagging finger, pointing, tapping, etc.,
    to give emphasis.
Helping = returning balls, setting up skittles, etc.
Rules and method = verbal orders concerned with the rules
    of the game and method of play.

The last category was chosen because some mothers seemed
especially concerned with organizing in this area, and it
was felt that it might be significant.

(3) Evidence of favouritism. Certain areas of the mother's
behaviour were considered from this point of view. They
were: smiles and laughs, positive speech, attending (watching or helping or playing with a child). Totals in these
categories received by our subject were compared with totals
received by the other (or the most favourite other) sibling
—they were expressed as a % of the totals for both children. Hence scores of over 50% indicated that our child was
favoured.

In all the Follow-up studies described above, analysis has followed the same pattern as in the nursery study. Children, moth-

ers and siblings have been ranked for totals (occasionally %s)
of items of interest and group differences assessed by the Mann-
Whitney U test.

In order to compare the families of our subjects, mothers and
siblings are labelled with the child's hostility group. This is
not entirely legitimate since a given mother may, for instance,
have children of different hostility groups. However, the distribution seems far from random and there is considerable evidence of differential treatment of children.

(4) Results and Discussion

It is not possible to give, in full, the results of this extensive investigation. Hence attention will be focused on some of
the more important findings; they will all be reported in more
detail elsewhere.

Little will be said of the Playground Observations apart from the
fact that the characteristics shown by the children at play are
very much in accord with the nursery school picture.

The Teacher Enquiries can be treated in more detail. The res-
ults for the Rutter Questionnaire and the Teacher Structured
Questions are presented (as in Table 3 of the nursery study) in
Tables 4 and 5.

The school results seem unambiguous in indicating that the Teasers and, to a lesser extent, the Teaser-specifics, are difficult
and even disturbed in their behaviour at school, while the Specifics and the Games group give no trouble. This is perhaps a
surprising result for the Games group but it may well be in line
with their timid, anxious-to-please behaviour outside a game
situation. The teachers did not see them in the playground.

Of the family investigations, the Behaviour Inventory and the
Tea-party will be given the most attention, although the other
enquiries will be referred to.

From the Behaviour Inventory results (Table 6), it can be seen
that, in contrast to the position at school, it is the Games
group who show behaviour problems at home. These children are
significantly higher than all others on overactivity, overtalk-
ativeness and sibling friction, and this contrasts with behaviour
observed in the nursery. They are also higher than most (all

except Teasers) in anxiety and unpopularity as judged by their
mothers.

It is of interest, too, that the Teasers do not tend to score
highly. This is surprising in view of their disruptive and often very hostile behaviour at nursery and at school. This will
be discussed later. Wolff also found no correlation between the
results of the Behaviour Inventory and the Rutter Questionnaire
for individual children although she did find that both methods
adequately distinguished her disturbed and normal samples.
Clearly some, but not all children behave differently at home
and at school.

It is also of interest that the Specifics are the only group to
show no signs of disturbed behaviour either at home or at school.

The Family Structured Interviews = Tea-parties provide a great
deal of information about relationships within the family. The
situation was clearly an artificial one and the mothers, in particular, wanted to give a good impression. This may account
for the fact that there were relatively few inter-mother differences in qualities such as warmth, nurturance, organizing severity; all were friendly and persuasive. However, they did differ in less obvious or less easily controlled qualities — negativity (provoked by their children), conversation, favouritism
and methods of control.

With few notable exceptions, the children were much less con-
strained than their mothers and many arguments and even fights
developed.

The results of (1) Speech analysis are given in Table 7. This
is a summary only of the significant differences between the
groups calculated on the basis of Mann Whitney U tests, as before. There is no space to present all the figures involved.

The most common and most highly significant outcome seems to be
that both the children and the mothers can be divided into two
sets — the Games group and the Teaser-specifics (1 and 3) on the
one hand and the Teasers and the Specifics (2 and 4) on the
other. Children of Groups 1 and 3 are highest in negative and
organizing speech, Groups 2 and 4 in positive speech and conversation. This dichotomy is the same as that revealed in the
Behaviour Inventory where children of Groups 1 and 3 appeared
as more difficult and disturbed than Groups 2 and 4. In this
respect, therefore, these two types of investigation validate
one another.

TABLE 4
Rutter Questionnaire

Scores greater than 9 indicate possible disturbance.

In lower line: 1 = Games group; 2 = Teaser; 3 = Teaser-specific; 4 = Specific.

Average score
2 teachers

13½-12½-12 -10½- 8 - 5½- 5 - 4½- 4½- 4 - 4 - 4 - 3½- 3 - 1½- ½- 0   2 > rest**
2 - 3♀- 2 - 2 - 2 - 1 - 3♀- 4 - 4 - 1 - 4♀- 3 - 4 - 2 - 1 - 4♀- 3♀

Highest score
any teacher

19 -13 -12 -11 -10 - 8 - 6 - 5 - 5 - 4 - 3 - 3 - 1 - 0   *2+3>1+4
2 - 3♀- 2 - 2 - 3 - 4 - 1 - 4♀- 4 - 4 - 39♀- 1 - 1 - 2 - 4♀- 3♀   p < 0.05

(Disagreement between teachers exceeded 2 points in 6 out of 17 children.)

There is thus a possibility of disturbance in 4/5 Teasers and 2/4 Teaser-specifics.

TABLE 5

Teacher Structured Questions

High scores indicate favourable qualities. Scores are averages for two teachers.

Work ability	15 -15 -14½-14½-14 -13½-13 -12½-12 -11½-10½-10 - 9½- 8½- 8 - 7	***4+1>3+2**	
	1 - 4 - 4♀- 4 - 4 - 3♀- 2 - 3♀- 2 - 4 - 1 - 3 - 3♀- 2 - 2 - 2	p < 0.01	
Popularity	5½- 5 - 4½- 4 - 4 - 4 - 4 - 4 - 3½- 3½- 3½- 3 - 2½- 1½	4+1>3+2**	
	4 - 4♀- 1 - 1 - 1 - 2 - 3♀- 3♀- 4 - 4 - 4 - 2 - 4 - 3♀- 2	p < 0.025	
Non-emotionality	11½-11½-11 -11 -10½-10 -10 - 9½- 9½- 9½- 9 - 8½- 8 - 8 - 7 - 6 - 5	2 < rest***	
	1 - 4♀- 3♀- 3♀- 3 - 1 - 1 - 4♀- 4 - 4 - 2 - 2 - 2 - 4 - 2 - 2 - 2		
Behaviour in class	21 -20 -19½-19 -19 -18 -18 -18 -17 -16½-16 -15½-14½-12½-12 - 9½	2 < rest***	
	1 - 3♀- 4♀- 1 - 3♀- 3 - 3♀- 4♀- 4 - 4 - 2 - 1 - 4 - 2 - 2 - 2		
Co-operative-ness and self-confidence	15 -14½-14 -14 -13½-13 -13 -12½-12 -12 -12 -11 -10½-10 -10 -10	2 < rest*	
	4♀- 4♀- 1 - 4 - 3♀- 1 - 2 - 3♀- 1 - 3 - 4 - 2 - 2 - 3♀- 2 - 2 - 4		

TABLE 6

Behaviour Inventory

Total scores for 25 behaviour traits. High scores indicate disturbance.

Total scores	64-49-45-44-44-43-42-41-40-38-36-31-30-30-29-27	**1+3>2+4**
	1 -1 -2 -3 -3º-1 -2 -2 -3º-4 -4º-2 -4 -3º-2 -4º-4	p < 0.025

TABLE 7

Analysis of Speech at Tea-Parties. Significant Differences
Between Families of Children of Different Hostility Groups.

Results represented as in Table 3 (see p. 38 for explanation).
Mann Whitney U test applied unless marked F (= Fisher's Exact Probability Test).
Group 1 = Games group; Group 2 = Teasers; Group 3 = Teaser-specifics; Group 4 = Specifics.

	Mother (M) all speech	Child (Ch) all speech	M - Ch	Ch - M	Child - Sibs	Sibs - Child
Positive speech %	N.S	* **4+2>3+1* p < 0.001	N.S	*4+2>3+1 p < 0.01	*4+2>3+1* p < 0.001	*2>1+3+4 p < 0.05
Positive tone of voice	N.S	* ***4+2>3+1 p < 0.025	N.S	*4>1+2+3 p < 0.05	4+2>1+3 p < 0.006	*2+4>1+3* p < 0.001

Conversation	*4>1+2+3 p<0.05	**4+2>1+3 p<0.001	*4>1+2+3 p<0.05	*4+2>1+3** p<0.01	**4+2>1+3** p<0.001	N.S
Nurturant speech	N.S	1+2+4>3* p<0.01	N.S	1+2+4>3* p<0.05	N.S	N.S
Organizing speech %	N.S	*3+1>4+2** p<0.01	N.S	1+3>2+4 p<0.025F	N.S	**3+1>4+2*F p<0.001
Organizing speech - totals	2+4>3+1* p<0.05	**1>2+3+4 p<0.025		1+3>2+4 p<0.05F	*3+1>4+2** p<0.027	**3+1>4+2** p<0.002
Competitive speech			*4+2>3+1** p<0.01	N.S	1+2+3>4* p<0.05	N.S
Attention seeking speech %				*3>1+2+4* p<0.05	N.S	N.S
Attention seeking tone of voice			*3+1>2+4** p<0.025	*3+1>2+4** p<0.025	1+3+4>2* p<0.05	1+3+4>2** p<0.001
Negative speech %	**3+1>2+4 p<0.01	***1+3>4+2** p<0.001	**1+3>2+4* p<0.01	**1+3>2+4* p<0.001	**1+3>2+4* p<0.001	**1+3>2+4 p<0.027
Negative tone of voice	1+3>2+4 p<0.001	1+3>4+2** p<0.001	*1+3>2+4 p<0.01	1+3>4+2** p<0.001	1+3>4+2** p<0.001	N.S

TABLE 8
Mother's Controlling Methods
(F = Fisher Exact Probability Test)

Manipulating totals - ½hr	10- 7- 7- 4- 3- 2- 2- 1- 1- 0- 0- 0- 0- 0- 0- 0	2 > rest*
	2- 2- 1- 2 1-3♀- 2-3♀- 4- 1- 2-3♀- 3-4♀-4♀- 4	4 < rest***
Physical control - ½hr	32-12-12-11- 9- 7- 5- 4- 4- 3- 2- 1- 1- 0- 0- 0	2 > rest*
	2- 2- 2- 1-4♀-3♀- 2- 3- 1-3♀-4♀- 4- 2- 1-3♀- 4	
Total help in games - ½hr	30-28-23-22-15-14-13-10- 9- 7- 7- 3- 3- 3- 3- 2	2 > rest**
	2-3♀- 2- 2- 1- 2- 1- 3- 2-3♀-4♀-1-3♀-4♀- 4- 4	4 < rest***
Total verb. org. rules & how - ½hr	55-21-20-16-13-10- 9- 8- 6- 6- 6- 5- 5- 2- 2- 1	2 > rest* F
	2- 2- 3- 1- 2- 2-4♀-3♀-1-3♀-4♀- 4- 4- 1- 2-3♀	

TABLE 9
Favouritism

% Child/Child + Sibling most favoured in family

% Smiles and laughs	*86-*83-*70- 60- 52- 45- 40-*40- 35-*32-*31-*26-*23-*0	****4+2>3+1*
	4♀- 4♀- 4 - 3♀- 2 - 2 - 2 - 2 - 3♀- 1 - 1 - 3♀- 3 - 1	p < 0.003
% Positive speech	*76-*75-*73- 53- 47- 46- 44- 43-*39-*31-*28-*22-*18	***4+2>3+1
	4♀- 3♀- 4♀- 4 - 2 - 2 - 2 - 3♀- 2 - 1 - 2 - 3♀- 1 - 3	p < 0.036
% Attending	72- 57- 57- 55- 53- 53- 46- 45- 43- 40- 38- 36- 35- 33	****4+2>3+1
	4♀- 4♀- 4 - 3♀- 3♀- 2 - 2 - 1 - 2 - 2 - 3♀- 3 - 1 - 1	p < 0.036

Taking the children group by group:
Games group (1) are the most negative and competitive and the
least positive in their speech;
Teasers (2) are the least negative and organizing;
Teaser-specifics (3) are the most organizing and the least con-
versational and nurturant;
Specifics (4) are the most positive and conversational.

Of relationships between other members of the family it can be
said that the conversational qualities of the Specifics extends
throughout the family. So does the negativity of the Games
group. But the differences in organizing speech apparent between the Teaser-specifics (high) and the Teasers (low) is mainly
an inter-sibling affair.

Mother's Controlling Methods. As can be clearly seen from
Table 8, the Teasers (Group 2) receive more than other children
of all these forms of control. In some cases this was so excessive as to leave the child almost no freedom of initiative
— almost every ball was bowled to order. Only one Group 2 child
is exceptional here (Colin). By contrast the Specifics were
often not organized at all. Frequently their mothers sat and
watched while the children improvised their own rules.

Favouritism. The evidence is given in Table 9. The figures
are % child/child+sibling in every case. Over 50% means our
subject is favoured. A * by the score means that the difference
between sibs is significant.

Clearly the Specifics (4) tend to be the most favoured and the
Games group (1) the least favoured members of their families.
Teaser-specifics (3) tend to be disfavoured with respect to a
much younger sibling, rarely with siblings nearer in age. Possibly this is not resented so much.

It is now possible to attempt a synthesis of all the family
study results as they throw light on the characteristics of the
hostility groups.

Group 1 = Games group. These are disfavoured members of their
families. At the tea-parties they were very negative and contrary and they received negative behaviour in return. The children argued among themselves and tried to dominate one another.
However, our child was not quite so negative in tone of voice
as in what he said. In fact, Group 1 boys significantly headed
a rank order for ambivalent speech (nasty remarks said in a nice
way).

From structured questions it appears that sibling friction with
many fights occurs commonly at home. Also, all mothers said
they found these overactive attention-demanding boys difficult
and all admitted a preference for siblings whom they found war-
mer and more responsive. Only one could describe interests in
common with her son. Instead, these boys have sporting interests and better contact (from Standard Day figures) with their
fathers than any other group.

It might be suggested that these children, feeling disfavoured
but desiring mother's affection, cover their hostility in a
friendly manner and find an ideal outlet for it in games situations. However, their tensions are seen in their anxiety, their
overactivity and their poor peer relationships. In addition,
all have had quite serious accidents when over three, including
taking aspirins, dog bites and breaking bones.

Group 2 = Teasers. The group is surprising in the contrast between difficult, hostile behaviour at school and apparent docil-
ity at home. However, at the tea-party they were distinguished
mainly for the absence of bad qualities rather than for the
presence of good ones.

During the games they seemed subdued and inhibited. They were
unnaturally nice to their siblings, they talked rather little
and there was little obvious enjoyment. This seemed in most
cases directly related to the fact that they were told exactly
what to do and how to do it.

From structured questions it seems that all these mothers (and
only one other) are especially concerned with manners, home
tasks, rules, appearance and cheekiness. Rules are enforced
strictly, often severely. They like their children for being
amenable, helpful and having good manners and appearance. On
the other hand, only one of these five boys goes out to any regular evening activity. The picture emerges of mothers more concerned that their children should be presentable and useful
rather than interested in them for their own sake.

Finally, fathers do not appear to have played a stable role in
the lives of these boys. One child is illegitimate and for the
others there have been long absences or periods when the father
was "too busy" or "not interested".

Group 3 = Teaser-specifics. The main characteristic of these
children in the nursery (and playground) was their bossiness and
their unfriendly speech. This was also apparent at the tea-
parties where they seemed contrary with their mothers, high in

organizing and attention-seeking speech and low in nurturance
and conversation. Bossiness and antagonism was even more apparent between the siblings and in two cases there were severe
quarrels. Mothers tried to be nice but the child's contrariness
often provoked negative speech. Often the friction was mainly
with one (usually older) child, although in most cases the mother
did not favour this child.

Structured questions support this picture. Many sibling fights
(often damaging) were reported. The mothers seem fond of our
child, however, they share activities with them and regard them
as interesting, good company, good natured and sociable. All
the children go to clubs.

In brief, these children seem to have supportive mothers but at
least one very unfriendly sibling (in three out of four cases
an older one). Relatively few workers have considered sibling
friction as a factor stimulating aggression but Patterson et al.
(1967) have argued how this could be so, particularly if the
mother does not intervene to make the behaviour less rewarding.
Family size tends to be larger in this group, hence these mothers might be too busy to attend to quarrels.

Group 4 = Specifics. All these children are friendly and un-
demanding. At the tea-parties the outstanding quality was conversation. It was shown by the whole family; there were many
jokes and much enjoyment. It parallels the self-oriented and
objective speech typical of them in the nursery. These children
were never disfavoured and tended to be favoured.

From Standard Day data we see that they score highest in independent activities and their mothers in nurturance (helping with
homework, playing with, reading to, etc.). Structured questions
show that discipline is significantly less severe (little physical punishment), that both parents share many interests with
their children and that, in particular, the fathers do things
other than sport with them (handicraft, drawing cartoons). All
go to clubs and all are good friends with their siblings in
spite of some quarrels.

Group 4 mothers are not especially warm. Some of them scored
low in rank orders of positive and nurturant speech and in hugs
and kisses. But they were highest in smiles and laughs. They
are friendly but not fussy.

In this study, as in the Nursery study, the random groups ABCD
were also tested for the possibility of chance correlations.
They yielded about a quarter of the correlations found for the
hostility groups and again no coherent picture emerged from them.

CONCLUSION

This study has shown that these 17 children, grouped in the nursery according to their dominant type of hostility, show behaviour differences which remain consistent at 7 - 8. Moreover, the group which seemed socially well adjusted in the nursery showed no sign of behavioural disturbance either at home or at school, whereas all the other groups did so in one or both of these situations. In addition, family difficulties have been demonstrated, which could be influential and which are different for each group.

The smallness of this sample allowed a considerable amount of data to be collected on each child. On the other hand it made rigorous statistical analysis difficult and hence it leaves open the query that the differences between the groups depend on factors other than the hostility characteristics which define them. Against this it can be argued that the nature of the behavioural and family characteristics of each group is in keeping with the nature of its dominant hostility type. Harassment is malicious, games hostility suggests concealed maliciousness; it is consistent that harassment specialists show signs of unfriendliness, games specialists of being "anxious to please". And it is plausible that overcontrolling by mother on the one hand and adverse favouritism on the other could stimulate these attitudes.

Whatever its shortcomings, this pilot study gives weight to the idea that different types of hostility do carry different implications and that a study of them might throw more light on the different effects of some background factors already known to influence aggression. Many of these may not be primary factors but a realization of their mode of influence may assist attempts to deal with aggressive behaviour.

ACKNOWLEDGEMENTS

M.M. is grateful to the Mental Health Foundation, the Social Sciences Research Council and to Professor Niko Tinbergen for financial support in this work. She would also like to thank her many assistants and advisors, the staff of the nursery and primary schools, the parents and the children.

REFERENCES

Barker, M. (1939) A technique for studying the social-material activities of young children, Monog. Soc. Res. Child Devel. 3.

Barker, R.G., Kounin, G.S. and Wright, H.F. (1943) Child Behavior and Development. New York and London, McGraw Hill.

Carpenter, C.R. (1965) The howlers of Barro Colorado Island, in DeVore, I. (ed.), Primate Behaviour: Field Studies of Monkeys and Apes, pp. 250-91. New York, Holt, Rinehart & Winston.

Davis, J.A. (1961) Compositional effects, role systems and the survival of small discussion groups, in Hare, A.P. et al. (eds.), Small Groups. New York, Knopf.

Douglas, J.W.B., Cooper, J.E., Lawson, A. and MacNeil, J. (1968a) A method for assessing family interaction and the activities of young children, Proc. R. Soc. Med. 61, 1319-1321.

Douglas, J.W.B., Lawson, A., Cooper, J.E. and Cooper, E. (1968b) Family interaction and the activities of young children. Method of assessment, J. Child Psychol. Psychiat. 9, 157-71.

Feshbach, S. (1964) The function of aggression and the regulation of aggressive drive, Psychol. Rev. 71, 257-72.

Feshbach, S. (1970) Aggression, in Mussen, P.H. (ed.), Carmichael's Manual of Child Psychology, Vol II. New York, Wiley.

Goodall, J. van Lawick (1968) The behaviour of free-living chimpanzees in the Gombe Stream Reserve, Animal Behav. Monog. 1, pt. 3.

Hall, K.R.L. and DeVore, I. (1965) Baboon social behaviour, in DeVore, I. (ed.), Primate Behaviour: Field Studies of Monkeys and Apes, pp. 53-110. New York, Holt, Rinehart & Winston.

Johnson, R.N. (1972) Aggression in Man and Animals. Philadelphia, Saunders & Co.

Kelly, G.A. (1970) A brief introduction to personal construct theory, in Bannister, D. (ed.), Perspectives in Personal Construct Theory. New York, Academic Press.

Kummer, H. (1968) Social Organisation of Hamadryas Baboons.
    Chicago University Press.

Lorenz, K. (1966) On Aggression. New York, Harcourt Brace.

McGrew, W.C. (1971) An Ethological Study of Children's Behav-
    iour. New York, Academic Press.

Patterson, G.R., Littman, R.A. and Bricker, W. (1967). Asser-
    tive behaviour in children. A step towards a theory of
    aggression in children, Monog. Soc. Res. Child Devel., 32(5),
    serial no. 113.

Piaget, J. (1959) The Language and Thought of the Child, 3rd
    ed. London, Routledge & Kegan Paul.

Rutter, M. (1967) A children's behaviour questionnaire for com-
    pletion by teachers: preliminary findings, J. Child Psychol.
    Psychiat. 8, 1-11.

Saayman, G.S. (1971) Behaviour of the adult males in a troup
    of free-ranging Chacma baboons (Papio ursinus), Folio Prim-
    atology, 15, 36-57.

Slater, P.E. (1955) Role differentiation in small groups, in
    Hare, A.P. et al. (eds.), Small Groups. New York, Knopf.

Smith, P.K. and Connolly, K. (1972). Patterns of Play and
    Social Interaction in Preschool Children, in Blurton Jones
    (ed.), Ethological Studies of Child Behaviour. Cambridge
    University Press.

Wolff, S. (1967) Behavioural characteristics of primary school
    children referred to a psychiatric department, Brit. J. of
    Psychiat. 113, 885.

EXPERIMENTS ON THE REACTIONS OF JUVENILE DELINQUENTS TO FILMED VIOLENCE

L. Berkowitz, R. D. Parke, J. P. Leyens, S. West and R. J. Sebastian

On March 13, 1969, a war film was shown aboard Trans World Airlines Flight 7 as it flew from New York to Los Angeles. Suddenly
one of the passengers became violent. The captain was called
and he tried to quiet the man but succeeded only in getting
punched. It took five other passengers plus the captain to sub-
due the troublemaker in a wild mêlée. Later, when he was questioned about this incident, the offender said, "I was watching
this war movie and saw everybody fighting, so I thought I would
start" (Toronto Globe and Mail, March 14, 1969).

Early in 1975 a freelance journalist interviewed the members of
a street gang in one of the roughest sections of New York City.
They talked about violence on TV. The leader, a teenager named
"Savage", was particularly fond of The Untouchables, a series
about a Treasury agent in Prohibition-era Chicago then being
re-run on one of the local channels. "It's got the action",
Savage explained. "A lot of shooting. Killing. Pushing people
off roofs ... I like violence." He didn't like to see rape portrayed on television, however. He claimed it gave many guys
the wrong ideas. "They go out and do it just for the hell of
it" (William Gale, in New York Times, March 30, 1975).

People can get all sorts of ideas. In 1973 a young woman was
assaulted by a gang of youths in Boston who poured petrol on
her and then set her afire. The Boston police were sure that

* A more complete report of this research can be found in Parke,
R.D., Berkowitz, L., Leyens, J.P., West, S. and Sebastian,
R.J., Film Violence and Aggression: A Field Experimental Analysis, in Berkowitz, L. (ed.), Advances in Experimental Social
Psychology, Vol. 10. New York, Academic Press, 1977. ·The
research reported in this paper was conducted under NIMH
grant MH17955 to Leonard Berkowitz and Ross D. Parke.

59

the hoodlums had copied a very similar scene shown just the day
before in a very popular TV crime program.

Here is one more illustration of this apparently media-induced
spread of violence. The television play Doomsday Flight, broad-
cast in the U.S. and elsewhere, told the story of an attempt to
extort money from an airline. A telephone caller in the movie
warns the airline officials that one of their planes then in
flight carried a bomb which was set to explode if the plane des-
cended below a certain altitude. If they paid him the money he
wanted, he would tell them where the bomb could be found. The
telecast triggered a number of very similar extortion attempts
both in America and abroad. Telephone threats warning of pressure bombs were made to Western Airlines and National Airlines
in the U.S. following the showing of this film. Shortly after
it was aired to Canada in July 1971, the same kind of threat
phoned in to a Canadian airline caused a transatlantic flight
to be diverted to Denver, Colorado. The caller had said the
bomb would go off if the plane dropped below 5000 feet and the
Denver airport was 5300 feet about sea level. In some cases
the threats were taken seriously enough so that the airlines
paid the money demanded by the extortionists. Qantas, Austral-
ia's international airline, paid half a million dollars on being
warned that a pressure bomb aboard a Hong Kong flight would explode when the plane came in for a landing. After a number of
such incidents the Federal Aviation Administration asked TV
stations around the country to refrain from showing the movie.
The FAA administrator explained, "Our great concern is that the
film might have a highly emotional impact on some unstable individual and stimulate him to imitate the fictional situation in
the movie" (Wisconsin State Journal, August 11, 1971).

I could go on and on, reporting one case after another in which
television or movie portrayals of violence had apparently influenced viewers to act violently themselves. These newspaper
accounts, however, certainly do not demonstrate unequivocally
that filmed violence heightens the audience's aggressiveness.
Seeking to provide such a demonstration, a number of researchers
have carried out laboratory experiments in which the subjects
are shown either an aggressive or nonaggressive scene and then
have an opportunity to punish someone else. The great majority
of these investigations have found that the movie viewers were
more punitive after seeing the aggressive film than after watching the neutral movie (cf. Goranson, 1970; Liebert, Neale and
Davidson, 1973).

But despite this agreement, some critics have questioned whether the laboratory results can be generalized to more natural settings (cf. the discussion in Parke et al., 1977). Many of the subjects in these experiments were university students, the critics noted, and the students might have acted in a way they believed the researchers wanted in order to curry favor. Moreover, the critics also claimed, the laboratory environment is a highly artificial one and the aggression measures typically do not at all resemble naturalistic aggression. What does the laboratory have to do with the behavior in the real world, they ask?

In order to confront these and other objections, several investigators have turned to field experiments. These studies present more or less typical movies to people in a naturalistic setting and then record the viewers' more or less free behavior. My colleagues and I have conducted one such investigation. Along with other researchers, we wanted to determine how people outside of a university laboratory would act after they saw violent films when they could behave aggressively or not and could display whatever aggression they showed fairly naturally.

RESEARCH PROCEDURE

Three experiments were carried out to determine if the results frequently obtained in relatively restricted laboratory situations with supposedly "artificial" measures of aggression would also be observed with more realistic forms of aggression in natural settings. These investigations employed teenage male juvenile delinquents living in cottages within minimum security institutions. However, two studies were in the United States, in Wisconsin more specifically, and one was in Belgium.

In each case the adolescents in all of the cottages were first observed for about a week to determine the boys' more or less usual level of aggressiveness in their interactions with their housemates. Then, after these baseline measurements, several typical commercial movies were shown, one each evening for five nights in a row. Half of the cottages in each experiment viewed highly aggressive films and the others watched much less violent ones. Twelve different aggressive movies and 13 nonviolent films were used over the three studies. Ratings made by the boys after each movie presentation clearly indicate that the intended differences were established; the aggressive films were generally regarded as much the more brutal, violent and

cruel than the neutral ones. In the first study the particular
non-aggressive films we used were also rated as less interesting
and exciting than their more aggressive counterparts, but this
difference was eliminated in the second experiment by a more
judicious selection of nonviolent movies. Then, after the five
days of controlled exposure to the films, the boys in each cottage were again observed during the following no-movie week
(after a weekend of no observations).

The aggression measures were the same in each experiment.
Trained observers went into each cottage in the afternoon or
after dinner. Following a previously established but random
schedule, each observer recorded what a certain youngster was
doing at the time in terms of 14 different categories, then went
on to another previously designated boy, and then a third one,
and so on. Each adolescent was observed twice each night for an
evening's total of three minutes. The categories referred to
several kinds of nonaggressive behaviors, such as being engaged
in nonaggressive interaction with others or keeping to oneself,
as well as to aggressive conduct. For simplicity, the aggressive categories were grouped together to form three main indices, one dealing with physical aggression only even though this
did not necessarily involve an attack on someone else, another
pertaining to all forms of interpersonal aggression whether of
a verbal or physical nature, and the third being the sum of all
aggressive categories, including threats and attacks on inanim-
ate objects as well as interpersonal aggression.

RESULTS

In general, although there are some differences in detail, all
three experiments demonstrated that the diet of aggressive films
stimulated the boys to increased aggression during the movie
week and in the following period as well. Some of this influence was clearly imitative in nature. The youngsters occasionally copied the physically aggressive actions displayed on the
screen, for example by imitating the boxing motions portrayed
by the actors in one of the movies. However, this was by no
means the only thing that happened; the teenagers in the violent films group also exhibited some kinds of aggression they did
not see in the movies. In the Belgian study, as a case in point,
verbal aggression was analysed separately from the other aggression measures and was found to have been significantly affected
by the films. All in all, the violent movies led to a rise in
various forms of aggression, physical and verbal, and with

greater or lesser resemblance to the violence shown on the screen. Figure 1 summarizes the results obtained with the interpersonal aggression index in Study 1, while the findings for the physical aggression measure in the Belgian experiment are given in Fig. 2.

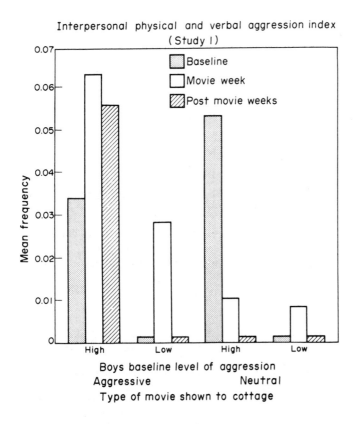

Fig. 1

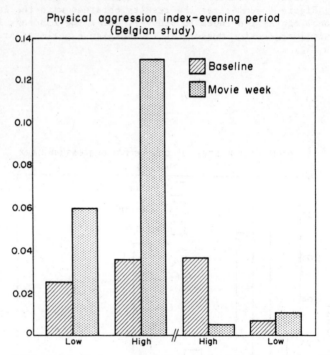

Fig. 2

This direct influence of the films was also apparent in laboratory observations made during the course of the two main American investigations. In both of these studies boys from the research samples were individually brought to a laboratory room
at the reformatory where they had an opportunity to be aggressive to a peer. In the first investigation along these lines
each teenager came to the laboratory supposedly to work on a
test of common sense with another boy, a stranger to him. As
he worked he was either strongly insulted by his partner who,
unknown to him, was actually the experimenter's accomplice, or

received only neutral remarks from this other person. Shortly
after this, the subject was given a chance to deliver electric
shocks to his partner as a judgement of the partner's performance on his task.

The results are summarized in Fig. 3. As is readily apparent,
we found that those people who had watched the violent movies
were now more punitive to the other boy than those who had seen
the non-aggressive films but only if they had been greatly provoked by him. Exposure to the week of filmed violence led to
stronger attacks on the boy who had just insulted them.

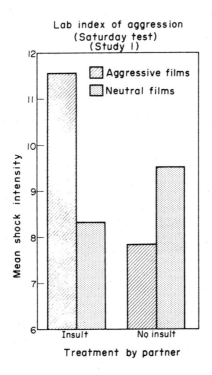

Fig. 3

This particular study obtained a significant effect for the
aggressive movies only when the subjects were angry. The second
experiment, on the other hand, found that the violent films
increased the aggression displayed by both angry and non-angry
people in the audience. In this investigation, which was conducted after the week of movie-viewing in our second study at the
reformatory, only verbal aggression was possible, not physical
attacks.

Briefly, on the day after the last movie each subject came to
the laboratory for a supposed study of problem solving under
stress. As he tried to complete the jig-saw puzzle given to him,
his partner—who again was the experimenter's confederate—was
required to distract him with a continual flow of chatter. Half
of the boys were mildly harassed by occasional bland remarks
such as "What did you do last night?". The others were severely
harassed by the confederate who peppered them with insults and
unfavorable comments. Following this treatment, each subject
had his turn to harass the confederate while that boy worked on
his puzzle. Here we found that the adolescents who had seen
the aggressive movies were much more hostile to the confederate
in their distracting comments to him than were their counterparts who had watched the neutral films. This occurred, furthermore, regardless of whether the boys had previously been severely
harassed by their partner.

Taken together, these two sets of results indicate that violent
films increase the chances that viewers will behave aggressively
even when they aren't angry. The viewers' anger facilitates
their aggression but isn't necessary. If they are somewhat rel-
uctant to attack an available victim strongly, and the only possible way of aggressing is to give him relatively painful electric shocks, the aggression-heightening influence of the violent
movie might not be readily apparent. This increased aggressiveness due to the films can be seen, on the other hand, if the
audience is not inhibited against aggression or if weaker forms
of aggression, such as verbal harassment, are possible.

But again notice that the subjects were not merely imitating
the actors on the screen. None of the movie characters admini-
stered electric shocks or verbally badgered someone else in the
way our subjects did. Violent films can give rise to a wide
variety of aggressive behaviors.

Questions still remain as to what kinds of people are most apt
to be affected by filmed violence. While recognizing the poten-

tially adverse consequences of movie and TV violence, the television industry in the United States has argued that only a few
violence-prone individuals will be spurred to attack others by
the aggression portrayed in the mass media. This is a misread-
ing of the actual evidence. First of all, as I mentioned earlier, scores and scores of experiments, some in laboratories
and others in more realistic settings, have demonstrated that
violent scenes often lead to heightened aggressiveness. There
obviously could not be so many studies with this result if only
a few violence-prone persons are affected. It is much more
accurate to say that many different kinds of people can be im-
pelled to increased aggressiveness by what they see — if they
are in the right frame of mind, if their inhibitions against
aggression are weak at the time, and if a suitable target is
available.

This summary statement is also supported by some of the findings
in our reformatory research. In our two main American studies
the teenagers were classified as having either a strong or weak
disposition to aggression on the basis of their behavior during
the base-line pre-movie period. We then compared the reactions
of these two groups of boys to the movies. By and large, both
types of youngsters were affected by what they had seen. Although they didn't react in exactly the same way, of course,
both the initially aggressive and less aggressive viewers exhibited more aggressive behavior following the violent movies than
after the less violent films. In Fig. 1, as a case in point,
you can see that the less as well as more hostile teenagers
displayed heightened interpersonal aggression soon after seeing
the aggressive movies. This film effect was obtained, furthermore, in the post-movie period as well as in the movie week in
our second study (which matched the two types of films better
on their interest and excitement for the teenagers). In the
Belgian experiment the cottages as a whole were classified as
high or low in aggressiveness during the baseline period. Figure 2 shows that the boys in both types of cottages became more
physically aggressive on seeing the violent films. Clearly,
viewers with weak as well as strong dispositions to aggression
can be stimulated to increased aggression by what they see.

Aggressive movies might heighten the instigation to aggression
but this won't always be revealed in open attacks. The viewers
might be unwilling to hurt anyone at that time. Perhaps they
think at that moment that it is wrong to injure someone. Or
maybe they are afraid that their potential victims are too powerful for them and will strike back if attacked. The Belgian

study divided the youngsters into those who had a dominant position in their cottages and those who were much less dominant,
as seen by their cottage mates. The dominant boys were the ones
who were most aggressive after the violent movies. Maybe they
felt freer to act out their film-induced aggressive tendencies
because their dominant status in the group protected them against
retaliation.

Our research has demonstrated so far that many of the aggressive
movies made today can heighten the audience's aggressiveness.
However, every violent film doesn't have this effect. Although
it is relatively uncommon, it seems to me, the movie might emphasize a kind of violence that the audience regards as horrible
or morally reprehensible. The film aggression therefore "turns
the viewers off", so to speak, and their inhibitions against
aggression are temporarily heightened.

We have seen this happen repeatedly with our university students.
The subjects in some six different experiments were more aggressive towards a person who had provoked them earlier if they had
watched "justified" aggression on the screen rather than an
incident of "less justified" violence.

In this research the filmed violence was usually defined as
justified or not by varying the information given the subjects
about the defeated character. Most of the experiments used an
excerpt from the movie Champion, in which the protagonist, a
champion prize fighter, took a bad beating during a title bout.
A brief synopsis provided before the movie started (supposedly
so that the subjects would better understand the scene) portrayed the champion in either a sympathetic or a less sympathetic
manner. In the latter case he was described as a person who had
frequently and shamelessly exploited other people in his rise to
the championship. The university students therefore generally
regarded the beating he received in the fight as justified punishment for his past misdeeds. In the opposing condition, by
contrast, the story summary depicted him more favorably and, as
a consequence, the students viewed his defeat as less justified
aggression.

Our question was whether juvenile delinquents would respond in
the same way as the university students employed in these earlier experiments. One could argue either way. Some authorities
contend that delinquents generally value being hard, tough and
able to outsmart others. These writers suggest that delinquent
boys are especially likely to think of social relationships as

hostile interactions   Presumably, they are greatly concerned
with their ability to exert power over their peers, and are also
likely to be exploitive, believing that they have the right to
take advantage of "suckers" (Hirschi, 1971). All in all, in the
words of some of these researchers, the delinquent boy seems to
be "sensitive to and aware of many ingenious techniques for
manipulating others. Rather than withdrawing from others, he
appears more oriented toward aggressively taking, demanding, and
doing" (Shore et al., 1967). We might expect from all this that
delinquents would not be unsympathetic to the tough, hard-hear-
ted exploiter — as the fight loser, the champion, is described
in the supposedly justified film aggression condition. They
might even be attracted to him. As a consequence, the beating
the champion received in the movie would appear relatively un-
warranted, and delinquents should, therefore, be less willing
to act aggressively themselves immediately afterwards. Following this reasoning, then, the difference between the "justified"
and "less justified" film aggression conditions found in the
earlier studies with university students should be minimized or
even reversed in the present delinquent population.

However, we should be careful not to exaggerate the uniqueness
of the values held by juvenile delinquents. Investigations have
also shown that these youngsters have many of the same beliefs
and values as their middle-class, normal counterparts. Much
like university students, they too could be affronted by the
fight loser's callous exploitation of other people and would,
therefore, also regard his beating as entirely proper and deserved. To the extent that this is the case, angry delinquent
boys viewing the presumably justified film aggression should be
more aggressive soon afterwards than other delinquents seeing
the less warranted violence.

This study employed 44 boys (median age 16 years) from the same
institution used in the field experiments. Summarizing the
procedure, in the first phase a partner evaluated the boys' answers to a series of simple questions by either belittling the
boy's answer (insult condition) or by providing innocuous, non-
evaluative feedback (non-insult condition). Then, in the next
phase, two-thirds of the subjects watched a 6½-minute film of
a prize fight from our standard movie Champion in which the
protagonist, Kirk Douglas, received a severe beating. As in
the earlier research, the scene was introduced by a synopsis
summarizing the story up to the fight. We used the same summary as before in which Kirk Douglas was said to be either a
scoundrel who had frequently exploited the people in his life

(justified aggression) or a much more sympathetic character
(less justified aggression). The remaining teenagers saw no
film. Next, for the measure of the boys' aggression, they were
permitted to choose among 10 levels of electric shock whenever
the partner, who had previously evaluated them, made an error
on a questionnaire. Each subject was given 10 opportunities to
shock his partner.

The principal finding concerns the heightened aggression displayed by the subjects in the insult-justified aggression condition. As in the experiments with university students, the
provoked boys who had watched the "bad person" being beaten
subsequently attacked their tormentor more severely than did
any other group (see Table 1). These juvenile delinquents evidently regarded the witnessed aggression in this condition as
being warranted or "proper" so that their own aggression also
seemed justified for the time being. Like the university students, they apparently thought an unfeeling exploiter of others
deserved a severe beating.

TABLE 1   Mean Intensity of Shocks Given to Confederate

	Film conditions		
	No film	Less justified film aggression	Justified film aggression
Neutral treatment	5.58abc (7)	6.40ab (7)	5.66abc (7)
Insult treatment	4.28c (7)	6.56ab (7)	7.70a (8)

Note: Cells having different subscripts are significantly dif-
        ferent, at the .05 level, by Duncan Multiple Range Test.

The numbers in parentheses are the number of cases in each cell.

The present results extend the generality of the earlier findings obtained with university students. In this sample as in
the university groups, when angry people watch a "bad" person
receive a beating, they are subsequently more inclined to attack
the "bad" individual in their own lives who had previously insulted them. These comparable results also suggest that the
delinquents in our sample had employed the same kind of moral

standards as did the university students in evaluating the defeated movie character; in both cases this character was evidently viewed as getting his "just deserts" if he had been depicted as someone who had ruthlessly exploited other people.

Moreover, the similarity in the pattern of results across the delinquent and non-delinquent populations suggests that our field study findings are probably not restricted to delinquent populations. Indeed, using different kinds of procedures with many different kinds of people, quite a few investigations have now demonstrated that media portrayals of aggression can increase the chances that people in the audience will act aggressively themselves.

REFERENCES

Berkowitz, L., Parke, R.D., Leyens, J.P. and West, S. (1974) Reactions of juvenile delinquents to "justified" and "less justified" movie violence, J. Res. Crime Delinq., 11, 15-24.

Goranson, R.E. (1970) A review of recent literature on psychological effects of media portrayals of violence, in Berkowitz, L. (ed.), Advances in Experimental Social Psychology, Vol. 5. New York, Academic Press.

Hirschi, T. (1971) Causes of Delinquency. Berkeley, Dal., University of California Press.

Liebert, R.M., Neale, J.M. and Davidson, E.S. (1973) The Early Window: Effects of Television on Children and Youth. New York, Pergamon Press.

Parke, R.D., Berkowitz, L., Leyens, J.P., West, S. and Sebastian, R.J. (1977) Film violence and aggression: A field experimental analysis, in Berkowitz, L. (ed.), Advanced in Experimental Social Psychology, Vol. 10. New York, Academic Press.

Shore, M.F., Massimo, J.L. and Moran, J.K. (1967) Some cognitive dimensions of interpersonal behaviour in adolescent delinquent boys, J. Res. Crime Delinq., 4, 243-247.

THE FAMILY BACKGROUNDS OF
AGGRESSIVE YOUTHS

D. P. Farrington

American research suggests that certain kinds of family environments are conducive to the development of aggression. Sears,
Maccoby and Levin (1957) interviewed nearly 400 mothers of 5-
year-old children, and concluded that children's aggression in
the home was related to the severity of punishment by the parents, the extent of disagreement between the parents, and the
lack of warmth of the mother. Bandura and Walters (1959) compared 26 aggressive youths aged 14-17 with 26 non-aggressive
youths matched for age, IQ, socio-economic status and area of
residence. In each case, they interviewed the mother, the father
and the youth independently. They found that the parents of the
aggressive youths were more likely to use physical punishment,
more likely to disagree with each other, and more likely to be
cold and rejecting.

McCord, McCord and Howard (1961) studied nearly 200 non-delinquent boys from the treatment group of the Cambridge-Somerville
study. Using records based on home visits by counsellors, psychiatric interviews, teachers' reports and other sources, cov-
ering the period from when each boy was aged 10 to when he was
15, they classified 25 of the boys as aggressive. They found
that the aggressive boys were likely to have punitive, rejecting
parents, who imposed erratic discipline, were in conflict with
each other, and did not closely supervise the boy. In another
research project, Eron, Walder, Toigo and Lefkowitz (1963) obtained peer ratings of the aggressiveness of children aged 8-9,
and compared them with interview responses made by each mother
and father. They found that the aggressiveness of the children
was related to the severity of the punishment imposed by the
parents.

These results, obtained in different studies, with children at
different ages, and with different operational definitions of
and methods of measuring aggressiveness and features of the family environment, are in remarkable agreement. They show that
cold, harsh, disharmonious parents tend to have aggressive children. However, since all the studies are essentially cross-
sectional and correlational, the chains of cause and effect are
far from clear. Consider the association between harsh physical

73

punishment by parents and aggressiveness of children. It may
be that this association reflects the tendency of children to
imitate the aggressive behaviour of their parents, or it may be
that aggressive children tend to elicit harsh treatment from
their parents. Another possibility is that there is no causal
link between harsh parental punishment and aggressive children,
and that the two only appear to be related because of the operation of a third factor. For example, it may be that harsh parental punishment and aggressive children are both more common
in low income families, and that this explains the association.
The only way to establish conclusively whether or not harsh punishment causes aggressiveness is to carry out an experiment in
which children are randomly allocated to parents with different
degrees of punitiveness, but this would be impossible in the
present ethical climate. Laboratory experiments designed to
study the effects of punishment (e.g. Parke, 1970; Wright, 1972)
use such artificial measures of punishment (e.g. a loud noise)
that it is difficult to generalize from them to real life.

When satisfactory experimentation is impossible, and when correlational research is inconclusive, perhaps the best hope for
answering causal questions is the longitudinal survey. In principle, longitudinal surveys can overcome many of the methodological problems of cross-sectional surveys, notably causal order
and retrospective bias (see Wall and Williams, 1970). Long-term
surveys are few and far between, because they are so difficult
to carry out, and this is especially true of surveys in which
aggressiveness is measured. Macfarlane, Allen and Honzik (1954)
followed up about 40 boys and girls from the Berkeley Guidance
Study from age 21 months to age 14 years, and obtained mothers'
reports of children's aggressiveness (temper tantrums) at different ages. Most of the inter-age correlations were significant, suggesting that aggressiveness is a relatively stable and
enduring personality trait. Aggressiveness at ages 5 and 10
correlated .42, and at ages 9 and 14 correlated .44. Tuddenham
(1959) reported an even higher correlation (.68) between ratings
of aggressive motivation at ages 20 and 33 for 32 men followed
up in the Oakland Growth Study.

Kagan and Moss (1962) obtained similar results in their follow
up at the Fels Research Institute of about 70 boys and girls
from birth to maturity. Their measures of aggressiveness were
based on observations in the home, interviews with the mother,
and interviews with the child. From birth to age 14, both
aggression towards the mother and physical aggression towards
peers were relatively stable. Only aggression towards the mother

significantly predicted verbal aggression in adults. An unusual negative result was obtained in Sears' (1961) follow up of his children at age 12. He found that aggression in the home at age 5 was not related to antisocial aggressive attitudes at age 12. However, the relationship between verbal aggression, aggressive attitudes and aggressive behaviour, even at the same age, is problematic. This paper will concentrate on aggressive behaviour.

The purpose of this paper is to present some results from a longitudinal survey carried out in England, called the Cambridge Study in Delinquent Development. This survey is primarily concerned with delinquency, but aggressiveness was measured at different ages, as were family background factors such as harsh discipline and parental disharmony. It is possible, therefore, to establish how far the family backgrounds of aggressive youths in England are similar to those of their American counterparts. It is also possible to establish the extent to which aggressive tendencies are stable over time in an English sample. Another question which can be investigated is the relationship between aggressiveness and delinquency, and the extent to which aggressive youths and delinquents have similar family backgrounds. Both in the present survey (West and Farrington, 1973), in another English survey (Mulligan et al., 1963), and in the American literature (e.g. Havighurst et al., 1962), it has been shown that aggressiveness predicts delinquency. McCord, McCord and Howard (1963) compared 26 aggressive delinquents with 25 aggressive non-delinquents and concluded that, while both groups had punitive, rejecting and disharmonious parents, the aggressive delinquents were more extreme in this respect, and were much more likely to have criminal or alcoholic fathers. In the present survey, Farrington and West (1971) compared 51 boys convicted before age 15 with 52 boys high on self-reported aggression up to age 14, and found that, while the two groups were similar in many ways, the delinquents were more likely to have disharmonious parents, and to have been separated from their parents.

THE PRESENT RESEARCH

As mentioned above, this research forms part of the Cambridge Study in Delinquent Development, which is a prospective longitudinal survey of a sample of 411 males. When they were first contacted in 1961 at age 8, they included all the boys in the second forms of 6 state primary schools in a densely populated working class area of London. They have now (up to the end of 1975) been followed up for about 14 years, and are aged about 22.

They were given batteries of tests in their schools when they
were aged 8, 10 and 14, and were interviewed at ages 16 and 18.
(These ages are approximate; the tests at age 8 were actually
taken at age 8-9, etc.)   Over the years, contact has been maintained with the vast majority of these boys. For example, at
age 18 it was possible to re-interview nearly 95% (389) of the
original sample of 411. Their parents were interviewed by
social workers about once a year from when the boys were 8 until
when they were 14, and their teachers filled in questionnaires
when they were 8, 10, 12 and 14. Information about the boys and
about their parents and siblings has also been obtained from
other sources, notably criminal, social and medical records.
Further details about this research project, and about the measures described below, can be obtained in West (1969), West and
Farrington (1973) and West and Farrington (1977).

Measures of the aggressiveness of each boy at ages 8, 10, 12 and
14 were derived from the teachers' questionnaires filled in at
these ages. The aggressive boys at ages 8 and 10 were those who
were nominated as being difficult to discipline. The aggressive
boys at ages 12 and 14 were those whose teachers gave them most
points for being disobedient, difficult to discipline, unduly
rough during playtime, quarrelsome and aggressive, over-compet-
itive with other children and unduly resentful to criticism or
punishment. Measures of aggressiveness at ages 16 and 18 were
derived from self-reports during the interviews at these ages.
The aggressive youths at age 16 were those who most frequently
admitted getting into fights, carrying and using weapons, and
fighting policemen. The aggressive youths at age 18 were those
who most frequently admitted getting into fights, starting
fights, and carrying and using weapons in fights.

A group of 27 violent delinquents was also identified, using
conviction records up to the end of 1974, when the majority of
youths were aged 21. A youth was only included in this group
if he had been charged with an offence that must have involved
violence against another person (such as causing actual bodily
harm), or if a police report said that he had used, or threatened to use, physical violence against another person during
the commission of an offence. The criteria for inclusion in
this group were quite strict. Robberies which merely involved
jostling or snatching were not counted, and neither was carrying an offensive weapon without actually using it or threatening to do so, nor threatening or insulting behaviour not involving violence. Almost all the 27 violent delinquents (24) had
been convicted for various degrees of violent assault or violent

robbery, and most of the violent offences occurred at age 17-18.
The remaining 98 youths who were convicted up to the end of 1974
were classified as non-violent delinquents. The violent delinquents tended to be multiple recidivists. Although only 3 of
them had more than one violent conviction, they had sustained
an average of 4.3 criminal convictions each, in comparison with
the average 2.7 convictions of the non-violent delinquents.

These indices of aggression and violence have been compared with
a variety of other factors measured at different ages. Family
income and marital disharmony were rated by the social workers
on the basis of the home interviews with the boys' parents when
the boys were aged 8, and marital disharmony was rated again
using interviews at age 14. The socio-economic status of the
family at ages 8, 10 and 14, on the Registrar General's scale,
was derived from information obtained in these interviews about
the current occupation of the family breadwinner. Family size,
defined according to the number of children born to a boy's
mother before his tenth birthday, was derived from interviews
with parents, from the boys themselves, from school records and
from outside agencies, including birth registrations at Somer-
set House. The boys from large families were those with 4 or
more siblings. The criminality of a boy's parents was assessed
from searches made at the Criminal Record Office. About a quarter of the boys (97) had one or both parents convicted before
their tenth birthdays.

A measure of parental attitude and discipline was derived from
the home interviews at age 8, combining the separate ratings of
mothers and fathers. Boys who were experiencing harsh parental
attitude and discipline were those whose parents were the most
extreme on ratings of cruel, passive or neglecting attitude,
erratic or very strict discipline, and harsh quality of discipline, implying cruelty or brutality of method. These factors
were all combined because they were so closely inter-related,
suggesting either that these aspects of child rearing behaviour
tended to occur together or that the social workers had found
it impossible to consider one in isolation from another. A
rating of parental supervision was also derived from the home
interviews at age 8, and the poorly supervised boys were those
whose parents were under-vigilant in watching over their activities or lax in enforcing rules of behaviour. A category of
nervous-withdrawn boys at age 8 was also derived from the parents' reports to the social workers, although in some cases
these reports were supplemented by information from medical
records. Temporary and permanent separations of a boy from his

parents up to his tenth birthday were assessed using the home
interviews and information from social agencies. Only those
whose separations had been caused by reasons other than death or
hospitalization (the most common of these other reasons being
desertion) were included in the separated group. This was because previous research (e.g. Douglas, Ross and Simpson, 1968)
and the present survey (West and Farrington, 1973) indicated
that separations caused by death or hospitalization had no del-
eterious effects. The measure of separations, therefore, reflects marital disharmony during the first 10 years of life.

The IQ of each boy at ages 8, 10 and 14 was obtained from the
Raven's progressive matrices tests given in the schools at these
ages. Vocabulary at ages 10 and 14 was measured using the Mill
Hill synonyms tests given in schools. Secondary school allocation at age 11, obtained from school records, was used as a
measure of educational achievement. The lowest group consisted
of boys in special schools for the educationally subnormal (a
small minority), boys placed in the lowest streams of secondary
modern schools or comprehensives, and, in the case of schools
which were not streamed, boys placed in the lowest positions of
their classes. All these indices of intelligence and attainment
were very significantly inter-related, suggesting that they were
all measuring the same concept, possibly scholastic failure.
The relative unpopularity of each boy at ages 8 and 10 was derived from peer rating tests given in schools. The daring of
each boy was assessed partly from the peer rating test at age
10, and partly from the reports of parents to social workers
when the boy was aged 8. Finally, the heights and weights of
the boys were measured in the schools, at ages 8, 10 and 14.

Whenever possible, the boys were dichotomized into the "worst"
quarter on each factor and the remaining three-quarters. This
was in the interests of comparability, so that, for example, it
was possible to investigate the relative importance of low income, large family size, low IQ and low vocabulary. For the
purposes of this paper, all the factors were classified into
those measured at ages 8-10, those measured at ages 12-14, and
those measured at ages 16-18. Where a factor had been measured
twice during a given age range, most often at ages 8 and 10,
the two measures were combined to produce a single measure. As
an example, 101 boys were isolated as the heaviest at age 8, and
102 at age 10. In these and other cases (e.g. height, IQ),
these figures were arrived at after correcting the raw figures
for the exact age on testing. These figures were then combined
to produce a group of 122 boys who were among the heaviest
quarter either at age 8, or at age 10, or at both ages.

THE MEASURES OF AGGRESSIVENESS

The major measures of aggressiveness used were the combined
teachers' ratings at ages 8 and 10, the combined teachers' ratings at ages 12 and 14, and the combined self-reports at ages
16 and 18. Each of these measures was obtained independently,
in the sense that the teachers who were rating at later ages had
no access to the earlier ratings by different teachers, while
the boys' reports were made without reference to their earlier
reports or to teachers' ratings. Table 1 shows that each of
these measures was significantly related to each of the other
measures, suggesting that aggressive tendencies are to some extent stable over time. As might perhaps have been expected,
the weakest relationship was between the aggressiveness measures
at ages 8-10 and 16-18. However, even in this case, the relationship was statistically significant. Furthermore, even the
most widely separated and different of the aggressiveness measures at single ages were significantly related. Eliminating
boys not known at either age, 36.4% of the 44 boys rated aggressive by their teachers at age 8 were among the 76 boys highest
on self-reported aggression at age 18, in comparison with 18.0%
of the remaining 334 rated (X^2 = 7.09 with 1 d.f., p < .01). In
other words, the boys who were nominated as difficult to discipline at age 8 tended to be those who were involved in fights at
age 18.

In an attempt to investigate aggressive careers, 400 boys were
studied who had aggressiveness scores in every one of the age
ranges, 8-10, 12-14 and 16-18. Figure 1 shows that, of the 311
boys with low scores at age 8-10, 77 had high scores at age
12-14. Of the 234 boys rated low at both 8-10 and 12-14, 47
were in the high aggressive group at 16-18. Nearly half of the
boys (187) were rated low at all three ages, while at the other
extreme 24 boys were rated high at all three ages. If a boy was
rated high at 12-14, whether or not he had also been rated high
at 8-10 did not help in predicting whether or not he would again
be rated high at 16-18. Thus, of the boys high at 12-14 and
high at 8-10, 45.3% (24 out of 53) were also high at 16-18, in
comparison with 46.8% (36 out of 77) of those high at 12-14 but
low at 8-10. On the other hand, if a boy was rated low at 12-14,
whether or not he had been rated high at 8-10 did help in predicting whether or not he would be rated high at 16-18. Thus,
of the boys low at 12-14 and high at 8-10, 33% (12 out of 36)
were also high at 16-18, in comparison with 20.1% (47 out of
234) of those low at 12-14 and low at 8-10. These results show
the extent to which past and present aggressive behaviour is

TABLE 1   Inter-relationships Among Measures of Aggressiveness

	Aggressive at 8-10 (93)	Aggressive at 12-14 (134)	Aggressive at 16-18 (119)	Violent delinquents (27)
Aggressive at 8-10 (93/317)		59.1/24.9**	40.4/26.7*	14.0/4.5*
Aggressive at 12-14 (134/277)			46.2/21.8**	14.3/2.9**
Aggressive at 16-18 (119/282)				15.1/3.2**

The figures in each cell give the percentage in each category on the row variable who fall into the extreme category on the column variable. * indicates that the two percentages are significantly different at p<.05 (based on the value of X^2 from a 2 x 2 table), while ** indicates that the two percentages are significantly different at p<.001. For example, 59.1% of the 93 boys rated most aggressive at 8-10 were also among the 134 boys rated most aggressive at 12-14, in comparison with 24.9% of the remaining 317 boys rated, a significant difference (X^2 = 36.7 with 1 d.f., p < .001).

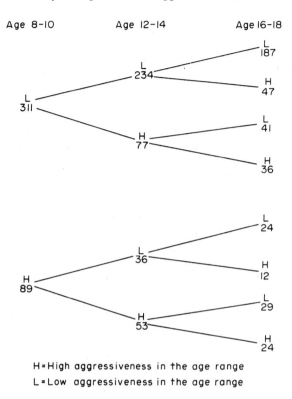

Age 8-10   Age 12-14   Age 16-18

H=High aggressiveness in the age range
L=Low aggressiveness in the age range

Fig. 1.   Aggressive careers

useful in predicting future aggressive behaviour, and suggest
that Markov models of aggressive careers might possibly be inappropriate (cf. Wolfgang, Figlio and Sellin, 1972).

The measures of aggressiveness at the three age ranges were
also significantly related to violent delinquency (see Table 1).
As might have been expected, aggressiveness at 8-10 was the
least closely related, although the relationship was still statistically significant (14% of those aggressive at 8-10 were
violent delinquents in comparison with 4.5% of the remainder;
$\chi^2 = 9.02$ with 1 d.f., $p < .005$). Turning the percentages round,
nearly half of the violent delinquents (48.1%) had been rated

aggressive at 8-10, in comparison with only 21.1% of the remainder. Aggressiveness at 8-10 was genuinely predictive of violent
delinquency, and, since only 3 out of the 27 violent delinquents
committed their violent acts before age 15, the measure at 12-14
can be considered predictive for all practical purposes. In
other words, teachers' ratings of aggressive behaviour in class
can predict future violent crime. The aggressiveness measure
at 16-18 is contemporaneous with most of the violent incidents.
The non-violent delinquents tended to be intermediate in their
aggressiveness between the violent delinquents and the non-delinquents. As an example, 70.4% of the violent delinquents,
49.0% of the non-violent delinquents, and 23.3% of the non-delinquents were among the aggressive group at 12-14.

THE PRECURSORS OF VIOLENT DELINQUENCY

Table 2 shows the relationships between the background factors
mentioned earlier and measures of aggressiveness. For example,
it can be seen that low family income and large family size
significantly predict whether or not a boy will become a violent
delinquent. An attempt was made to go beyond the gross relationships seen in Table 2 and to investigate the extent to which
factors were related to aggressiveness independently of other
factors. Low family income and large family size were closely
related to each other (in the 2 x 2 table, X^2 = 83.3, p < .001),
no doubt at least partly because the social workers took into
account the number of children in the house in rating the ade-
quacy of family income. Are low family income and large family
size related to violent delinquency independently of each other?
In order to test this, the partial ϕ correlations were used.
In a 2 x 2 table based on 400 boys, X^2 = 3.84 (the p = .05 level
of significance) corresponds to ϕ = .098, and X^2 = 10.83 (the
p = .001 level of significance) corresponds to ϕ = .165. The
significance levels for partial ϕ correlations (derived from the
F statistic) are very similar, a partial ϕ = .098 corresponding
to p = .05 and a partial ϕ = .163 corresponding to p = .001.

Low family income correlated .126 with violent delinquency, and
large family size .114. Both of these ϕ correlations are statistically significant, of course, reflecting the significant
values of X^2 indicated in Table 2. The ϕ correlation between
low family income and large family size was much greater at .450.
Controlling for family size, the partial ϕ correlation between
low family income and violent delinquency was .084, not statistically significant. Similarly, controlling for family income,

the partial ϕ correlation between large family size and violent delinquency was .065, not statistically significant. Therefore, it was concluded that low family income and large family size were not independently related to violent delinquency. Since the correlation and partial correlation for low family income were both higher than for large family size, it can be suggested that large family size only appeared to be related to violent delinquency because of its association with low family income, which was the more important factor. This kind of partial correlation analysis was repeated with all the background factors.

The factor which was most closely related to violent delinquency was harsh parental attitude and discipline at age 8. In fact, this was more closely related to violent delinquency than the aggressiveness measure at 8-10. Table 2 shows that 14.0% of those receiving harsh parental attitude and discipline became violent delinquents, in comparison with only 3.6% of the remainder ($\chi^2 = 12.3$, $p < .001$). Turning the percentages round, 61.5% of the violent delinquents had received harsh parental attitude and discipline, in comparison with only 27.1% of the remainder. Of the other family environment factors, criminal parents and separations both significantly predicted violent delinquency, and poor parental supervision and marital disharmony at 14 would have been significantly related to it if the numbers had permitted valid χ^2 tests. The ϕ correlations were .154 for poor parental supervision and .149 for marital disharmony. On the basis of the partial ϕ correlations, each of these five family environment factors was significantly related to violent delinquency independently of all the other factors. Furthermore, they were all related to violent delinquency independently of low family income, but low family income was not related to violent delinquency independently of poor parental supervision, separations or marital disharmony at 14. It seems plausible to suggest that low family income only appears to be related to violent delinquency because of its association with one or more of these other factors.

Of the other background factors, the assessment of daring at 8-10 significantly predicted violent delinquency. Daring was related independently of all other factors, and all the other factors were related independently of daring. Finally, the two measures of low IQ (at 8-10 and at 14) were significantly related to violent delinquency. Once again, each was related independently of all the other factors, and vice versa. Nor surprisingly, the two IQ measures were not significantly related independently of each other, since they are both essentially

D.P. Farrington

TABLE 2   The Backgrounds of Aggressive Youths

	% Violent delinquents out of whole sample (27/408)	% Aggressive at 8-10 out of whole sample (93/410)	% Aggressive at 16-18 out of whole sample (119/401)	% Aggressive at 16-18 out of those not aggressive previously (47/234)
Social background				
Low socio-economic status at 8-10 (168/243)	7.7/5.8	25.0/21.1	28.3/30.6	17.7/21.7
Low socio-economic status at 14 (121/258)	8.3/6.3	20.7/23.7	28.0/31.9	17.6/21.9
Low family income at 8 (93/318)	12.9/4.8*	31.2/20.2*	41.9/26.0*	32.6/17.3*
Large family size at 10 (99/312)	12.1/4.9*	22.2/22.8	39.4/26.5*	30.2/17.1
Family environment				
Harsh parental attitude and discipline at 8 (116/275)	14.0/3.6**	31.3/18.5*	37.7/25.7*	25.4/17.1
Poor parental supervision at 8 (74/309)	15.1/4.6†	28.4/20.8	45.2/25.1*	30.6/17.3
Marital disharmony at 8 (89/284)	10.2/5.7	31.8/19.0*	35.6/27.0	26.2/17.7
Marital disharmony at 14 (60/266)	15.0/4.5†	30.0/18.9	42.4/25.1*	40.6/16.0*
Separated from parent before 10 (90/321)	14.4/4.4*	32.6/19.9*	34.4/28.3	18.6/20.4
Criminal Parent before 10 (97/314)	14.4/4.2**	30.9/20.1*	42.1/25.8*	34.0/16.6*

Personality

Daring at 8-10 (121/287)	13.2/3.9*	40.5/15.0**	44.2/23.7**	27.7/18.3
Nervous-withdrawn at 8 (95/294)	5.4/6.8	13.8/24.8*	23.9/30.9	16.9/20.6
Unpopular at 8-10 (126/269)	8.8/4.9	26.2/20.8	35.5/25.8	20.6/19.9

Physical characteristics

Tall at 8-10 (161/248)	6.8/6.5	19.4/25.0	33.1/27.3	22.2/18.7
Tall at 14 (99/305)	8.1/5.9	17.2/24.7	32.7/28.9	17.2/21.5
Heavy at 8-10 (122/288)	7.4/6.3	17.2/25.1	26.7/31.1	14.7/22.8
Heavy at 14 (95/287)	6.3/6.3	16.8/24.1	30.1/29.1	20.0/19.9

Intelligence and attainment

Low matrices IQ at 8-10 (103/308)	13.7/4.2*	26.2/21.5	40.0/26.2*	26.2/18.8
Low matrices IQ at 14 (118/287)	12.7/4.2*	34.7/17.8**	36.8/26.9	28.3/18.4
Low Mill Hill vocabulary at 10 (124/277)	8.9/5.4	33.3/18.8*	37.4/26.4*	22.2/19.5
Low Mill Hill vocabulary at 14 (93/313)	10.8/5.4	29.0/20.8	39.6/26.7*	20.0/20.3
Low secondary school allocation at 11 (121/290)	8.3/5.9	31.7/19.0*	36.4/26.9	24.0/19.0

The figures in each cell give the percentage in each category on the row variable who fall into the extreme category on the column variable. * indicates that the two percentages are significantly different at p < .05 (based on the value of X^2 from a 2 x 2 table), while ** indicates that the two percentages are significantly different at p < .001. († indicates that the numbers are too small to carry out a valid X^2 test). For example, 12.9% of the 93 boys who were in low income families at age 8 were among the violent delinquents, in comparison with 4.8% of boys not in low income families, a significant different ($X^2 = 6.44$ with 1 d.f., p < .025). Boys rated 0 (not known or not applicable) on either variable are excluded in calculating these percentages.

measuring the same concept and were highly inter-correlated
(ϕ = .483). None of the other factors, including low socio-
economic status, unpopularity, height, weight and low educational
achievement, was significantly related to violent delinquency.
The violent delinquents, therefore, did not tend to be drawn
from the tallest and heaviest boys.

A search was also made, using partial ϕ correlations, for the
masking of relationships. As an example, nervous-withdrawn personality was very significantly related to harsh parental attitude and discipline (ϕ = .265), which in turn was more significantly related to violent delinquency than any other factor
(ϕ = .178). If there was no true relationship between nervous-
withdrawn personality and violent delinquency, the operation of
harsh parental attitude and discipline as an intervening variable would produce an artefactual observed correlation between
nervous-withdrawn personality and violent delinquency of .047.
The observed correlation was in fact -.013, and the partial correlation between nervous-withdrawn personality and violent delinquency, controlling for harsh parental attitude and discipline,
came to -.063. This suggests that the true negative relationship between nervous-withdrawn personality and violent delinquency was being masked by the positive correlations between
nervous-withdrawn personality and harsh parental attitude and
discipline, and between harsh parental attitude and discipline
and violent delinquency. However, none of the partial correlations emerging from these kinds of analyses reached statistical
significance.

To summarize, 6 factors measured at 8-10 predicted violent delinquency independently of every other background factor, namely
harsh parental attitude and discipline, criminal parents, poor
parental supervision, separations, daring and low IQ. Marital
disharmony at age 14 was also independently related. Furthermore, each of these factors was related to violent delinquency
independently of the measures of aggressiveness at 8-10, 12-14
and 16-18, just as the measures of aggressiveness were related
to violent delinquency independently of each of the background
factors. From an early age, then, the violent delinquents tended to have cold, harsh, disharmonious, poorly supervising and
criminal parents, tended to have low IQs, and tended to be rated
daring and aggressive.

A COMPARISON BETWEEN VIOLENT AND NON-VIOLENT DELINQUENTS

It was mentioned earlier that the non-violent delinquents tended to be intermediate in aggressiveness between the violent delinquents and the non-delinquents. To what extent do they share these background factors? Harsh parental attitude and discipline was the only factor which significantly differentiated between violent and non-violent delinquents. Nearly twice as many of the violent delinquents received harsh parental attitude and discipline (61.5% as opposed to 32.6%; X^2 = 5.92 with 1 d.f., p < .025). Furthermore, the non-violent delinquents did not differ significantly from the non-delinquents on this factor. Because of the smaller numbers involved in comparing 27 violent and 98 non-violent delinquents, a much stronger relationship than before (ϕ = .175) was required in order to achieve a statistically significant discrimination. Low IQ at 8-10 and separations nearly discriminated significantly between violent and non-violent delinquents (ϕ = .163 and .161 respectively) and both did not quite discriminate significantly between non-violent delinquents and non-delinquents. On the other hand, criminal parents, daring, poor parental supervision and marital disharmony at 14 all discriminated significantly between non-violent delinquents and non-delinquents, and did not discriminate between violent and non-violent delinquents to the same extent.

To summarize, just as the non-violent delinquents were intermediate in aggressiveness between the violent delinquents and the non-delinquents, they also tended to be intermediate in their possession of background characteristics. The greatest difference between the violent and non-violent delinquents lay in the fact that the violent delinquents were far more likely to have experienced cold, harsh parents, and they were also more likely to have had early separations from their parents and low IQs.

THE BACKGROUNDS OF AGGRESSIVE BOYS

Most of the background factors which were related to violent delinquency were also significantly related to aggressiveness at 8-10. It might be suggested that these factors had already exerted their aggression-producing effects by age 8-10, and that they were only related to violent delinquency because, as boys matured, there was a logical progression from aggressiveness in the primary school to violent delinquency. Table 2

shows that harsh parental attitude and discipline, criminal
parents, separations, low family income, daring and low IQ at
14 were all significantly related to aggressiveness at 8-10.
Perhaps rather surprisingly, low IQ at 8-10 was not significantly
related. Marital disharmony at 8, Mill Hill vocabulary at 10,
and low secondary school allocation at 11 were also significantly
related, as was nervous-withdrawn personality (negatively). Of
the social background and family environment factors, harsh
parental attitude and discipline was again and most closely related to aggressiveness. Judging from the partial correlations,
low family income, criminal parents and marital disharmony at 8
only appeared to be related to aggressiveness because of their
association with the more important factor of harsh parental
attitude and discipline. On the other hand, separations were
related independently of harsh parental attitude and discipline,
and vice versa.

Three of the measures of intelligence and attainment were significantly related to aggressiveness at 8-10. Low Mill Hill vocabulary at 10 and low secondary school allocation at 11 were not
related independently of low IQ at 14, suggesting that it was
reasonable to take low IQ as the most important factor. Daring
was related independently of all other factors, and this may be
because it is measuring much the same thing as aggressiveness.
The peer rating of daring may have been greatly influenced by
the rebellious behaviour of boys in their primary school classrooms. Nervous-withdrawn personality was also related to aggressiveness independently of all other factors, and again it may be
measuring much the same concept, but at the opposite end of the
continuum. As before, the negative correlation between nervous-
withdrawn personality and aggressiveness was considerably increased after partialling out the masking influence of harsh parental attitude and discipline (from -.106 to -.148). It may be
that aggressiveness and nervousness are two alternative reactions
to harsh parental attitude and discipline.

In view of the overlap between the different measures of aggressiveness, it was hardly surprising to find similar relationships
between aggressiveness and background factors at the later ages.
The figures for age 12-14 are not shown in Table 2, but all the
measures of intelligence and attainment, separations, daring and
nervous-withdrawn personality (negatively) were significantly
related to aggressiveness at this age. The figures for age
16-18 are shown in Table 2, and it can be seen that harsh parental attitude and discipline, poor parental supervision, marital
disharmony at 14, criminal parents, daring and low IQ were all

significantly predictive of aggressiveness at this age.

It is interesting to enquire which factors predicted the emergence of aggressiveness <u>for the first time</u> at later ages, and this is shown for age 16-18 in the final column of Table 2. When those who were rated aggressive at either 8-10 or 12-14 were eliminated, the only factors which significantly, and independently, predicted aggressiveness at 16-18 were marital disharmony at 14 and criminal parents. Low family income was not related independently of marital disharmony at 14. Of course, as the total numbers involved decrease, a stronger relationship is required in order to achieve statistical significance.

This applies with even more force in an analysis which was designed to investigate which factors would predict, out of those rated aggressive at 8-10, which boys would go on to be rated aggressive at all three ages. The most significant predictor was separations. Of the 24 boys rated aggressive at all three ages, 54.2% had been separated up to age 10, in comparison with 24.6% of the 65 boys rated aggressive at 8-10 but not at all three ages ($X^2 = 5.69$ with 1 d.f., p < .025). Perhaps rather surprisingly, the only other significant predictor of this was unpopularity. The unpopular boys among those who were aggressive at 8-10 tended to go on to be aggressive at all three ages. This result was not artefactually created by an association between separations and unpopularity.

In previous work on this longitudinal survey, attempts have been made to investigate causal questions about the effects on delinquency of attending different secondary schools (Farrington, 1972), of having criminal parents (Farrington, Gundry and West, 1975), and of being convicted (Farrington, 1977). It had been hoped that the results obtained here would help to elucidate the chain of cause and effect between family environment and child aggressiveness. Unfortunately, the fact that somewhat consistent aggressive tendencies were already apparent at age 8-10, when the family environment factors were first measured, meant that measures of the "dependent" variable of child aggressiveness were not, in general, available both before and after measures of the "independent" variables of family environment. The exception to this was marital disharmony, which was measured both at age 8 and at age 14. Marital disharmony at 14 proved to be the best predictor of newly emerging aggressiveness at 16-18. Furthermore, although the numbers were small, the indications were that newly emerging marital disharmony at 14 was followed by newly emerging aggressiveness at 16-18. Considering

only boys who were not rated aggressive at either 8-10 or 12-14
and whose parents were not rated disharmonious at 8, 6 out of
the 14 with disharmonious parents at 14 became aggressive at
16-18 (42.9%), in comparison with 23 out of the 142 whose parents
were not rated disharmonious at 14 (16.2%). These results are
in agreement with the hypothesis that marital disharmony causes
aggressiveness, although it is still possible that some other
unmeasured factor associated with marital disharmony was the
true causal agent.

CONCLUSIONS

The results given in this paper show that violent delinquents,
most of whose violent offences occurred when they were aged 17-
18, tended to be among the more aggressive from age 8 onwards.
At age 8-10, they tended to have cold, harsh, disharmonious,
poorly supervising and criminal parents. They also tended to
have low IQs and to be rated daring. They differed especially
from non-violent delinquents in having experienced cold, harsh
parents more often. Much the same constellation of background
factors was characteristic of those who were rated aggressive
at 8-10 and at later ages, and some of the factors (notably
criminal parents and later marital disharmony) predicted the
emergence of aggressiveness at 16-18. One possible interpretation of these results is that the factors which predispose
children to aggressive behaviour also tend to predispose young
adults to criminal violence.

These results agree with American researches in showing that
aggressive children develop in cold, harsh, disharmonious family environments. They also agree in their indication that
aggressiveness is a somewhat stable personality trait, at least
between ages 8 and 18. They also point to the independent importance of other factors, notably poor supervision, low IQ and
criminal parents. It is not easy to relate these results to
theories about the development of aggression. For example, the
modelling theory outlined by Bandura and Walters (1963) might
explain some of the results but not others. It would explain
why harshly punitive parents should tend to have aggressive
children, because children are said to imitate the aggressive
behaviour of their parents. However; the way in which this
theory might explain the relationship between low IQ and aggressiveness is not clear.

One problem is that the results obtained in a longitudinal sur-

vey such as this represent gross relationships between variables
at the end of long causal chains. Perhaps what is needed to
fill in some of the intervening links in each chain is a series
of careful observational studies in which minute elements of
parental behaviour are related to minute elements of child behaviour (see, for example, Lytton, 1971). Experimental studies
are also useful for this purpose, providing that the operational
definitions of the variables are not too divorced from real life.
In any investigation of the development of aggressive tendencies
over a number of years, it will be necessary to simplify the
true situation and measure only a limited number of factors. It
is to be hoped that a future long-term survey, concerned specifically with the development of aggression from birth to maturity, would include more frequent measurements and more extensive
analyses and operational definitions of different types of aggressive behaviour and of different aspects of child rearing, than
was the case in the present survey. However, such long-term
surveys raise enormous practical difficulties. A combination
of methods, from the small scale observational study dealing
with minute elements of behaviour to the large scale longitudinal
survey dealing with gross behavioural tendencies, is required
to test theories of the development of aggressiveness, and to
establish the causes of aggressive behaviour in children and
criminal violence in adults.

REFERENCES

Bandura, A. and Walters, R.H. (1959) Adolescent Aggression.
New York, Ronald Press.

Bandura, A. and Walters, R.H. (1963) Social Learning and Personality Development. New York, Holt, Rinehart & Winston.

Douglas, J.W.B., Ross, J.M. and Simpson, H.R. (1968) All Our
Future. London, Peter Davies.

Eron, L.D., Walder, L.O., Toigo, R. and Lefkowitz, M.M. (1963)
Social class, parental punishment for aggression, and child
aggression, Child Dev., 34, 849-867.

Farrington, D.P. (1972) Delinquency begins at home, New Soc.,
21, 495-497.

Farrington, D.P. (1977) The effects of public labelling, Br. J.
Crim. 17 (in press).

Farrington, D.P., Gundry, G. and West, D.J. (1975) The familial transmission of criminality, Medicine Sci. Law, 15, 177-186.

Farrington, D.P. and West, D.J. (1971) A comparison between early delinquents and young aggressives, Br. J. Crim. 11, 341-358.

Havighurst, R.J., Bowman, P.H., Liddle, G.P., Matthews, C.V. and Pierce, J.V. (1962) Growing up in River City. New York, Wiley.

Kagan, J. and Moss, H.A. (1962) Birth to Maturity. New York, Wiley.

Lytton, H. (1971) Observation studies of parent-child inter-action: a methodological review, Child Dev. 42, 651-684.

Macfarlane, J.W., Allen, L. and Honzik, M.P. (1954) A Developmental Study of the Behavior Problems of Normal Children between 21 months and 14 years. Berkeley, University of California Press.

McCord, J., McCord, W. and Howard, A. (1963) Family interaction as antecedent to the direction of male aggressiveness, J. Abnorm. Soc. Psychol. 66, 239-242.

McCord, W., McCord, J. and Howard, A. (1961) Familial correlates of aggression in non-delinquent male children, J. Abnorm. Soc. Psychol. 62, 79-93.

Mulligan, G., Douglas, J.W.B., Hammond, W.A. and Tizard, J. (1963) Delinquency and symptoms of maladjustment, Proc. Roy. Soc. Med. 56, 1083-1086.

Parke, R.D. (1970) The role of punishment in the socialization process, in Hoppe, R.A., Milton, G.A. & Simmel, E.C. (eds.), Early Experiences and the Processes of Socialization. New York, Academic Press.

Sears, R.R. (1961) Relation of early socialization experiences to aggression in middle childhood, J. Abnorm. Soc. Psychol. 63, 466-492.

Sears, R.R., Maccoby, E.E. and Levin, H. (1957) Patterns of Child Rearing. Evanston, Illinois, Row, Petersen.

Tuddenham, R.D. (1959) The constancy of personality ratings over two decades, Gen. Psychol. Mono. 60, 3-29.

Wall, W.D. and Williams, H.L. (1970) Longitudinal Studies and the Social Sciences. London, Heinemann.

West, D.J. (1969) Present Conduct and Future Delinquency. London, Heinemann.

West, D.J. and Farrington, D.P. (1973) Who Becomes Delinquent? London, Heinemann.

West, D.J. and Farrington, D.P. (1977) The Delinquent Way of Life. London, Heinemann (in press).

Wolfgang, M., Figlio, R.M. and Sellin, T. (1972) Delinquency in a Birth Cohort. Chicago, University of Chicago Press.

Wright, D. (1972) The punishment of children: a review of experimental studies, J. Moral Educ. 1, 221-229.

FAMILY, AREA AND SCHOOL INFLUENCES IN THE GENESIS OF CONDUCT DISORDERS

M. Rutter

Aggression can take many different forms and it would be unwise to assume that all varieties mean the same thing or have the same causes. Aggressive acts may be undertaken by normal individuals who show no signs of psychiatric disorder or of any other kind of psychopathology. On the other hand, persistently aggressive behaviour may sometimes constitute part of a more widespread disorder of conduct, as shown by numerous studies (see West, 1967; Robins, 1966; Quay, 1972). In these cases, the aggression may take the form of fighting, bullying, violent assault or destructiveness. Often it is associated with serious disturbances in personal relationships.

In disentangling the origins of these forms of behaviour there is a double research problem. First, why has the individual got a socially handicapping conduct disorder? and second, why does the conduct disorder take the particular form of aggressive acts? Both questions are important, but it is necessary to appreciate that they are not the same question and that quite different aetiological influences may be operating in the two cases.

This paper is solely concerned with the first question of the origins of conduct disorders and not at all with why the disorders involve aggressive acts. In the studies which are discussed some of the children with conduct disorders were seriously aggressive, but many were not.

OUTLINE OF STUDIES

The data which form the basis of this paper come from a series of detailed epidemiological enquiries undertaken with colleagues over the last 10 years (see Rutter et al., 1977; Rutter, 1977a). Most involved studies of the family in which detailed and sensitive interviewing techniques of demonstrated reliability and validity were used to investigate family life and relationships in its various forms (Brown and Rutter, 1966; Rutter and Brown, 1966; Quinton, Rutter and Rowlands, 1976). Attention was paid in the interviews both to what people reported and also to how they behaved with respect to attitudes, feelings and emotions.

Two different kinds of measure were used to assess children's
behaviour. First, scores on a behavioural questionnaire completed by teachers were used to determine whether or not children
were "behaviourally deviant". The questionnaire has been ex-
tensively tested and is known to have satisfactory reliability
and validity (Rutter, 1967; Rutter, Tizard and Whitmore, 1970;
Rutter et al., 1975a). A high (deviant) score on the questionnaire is significantly associated with the presence of psychiatric disorder as assessed by independent detailed interviewing
of parents, teachers and children.

Second, an individual clinical diagnosis of "psychiatric disorder" was made on the basis of a systematic and detailed parental
account of the child's behaviour as well as on information from
teachers (Rutter, Tizard and Whitmore, 1970; Rutter et al.,
1975a). Again, the ratings have been shown to be reliable and
to differentiate psychiatric clinic children from children in
the general population.

Information on school characteristics was obtained from the
schools themselves. The data included items such as extent of
teacher turnover and pupil absenteeism.

Reference will be made to four epidemiological studies, all but
one of which involved the investigation of random samples of
the general population. The one exception concerns a representative sample of all the families living in a particular geographical area, in which one or both parents had been newly
referred to a psychiatric clinic over a specified period of
time, and in which there was at least one child under the age
of 15 years (Rutter, 1970, 1971). The second study concerned
all 10-year-old children living on the Isle of Wight who attended state schools, and the third was a similar study of 10-
year-old children in one inner London borough (Rutter et al.,
1975a). The fourth study involved the same group of London
children and consisted of a systematic follow-up study into the
third year of secondary school at age 14-15 years (Rutter, 1977c;
Yule and Rutter, 1977).

As the investigations have been previous described in published
papers, no further details will be given here. Instead, the
paper will use research findings from the four studies to consider principles and issues with respect to family influences,
area differences, school differences and ameliorating factors.

FAMILY INFLUENCES

In the studies of 10-year-old children on both the Isle of Wight
and in inner London, various indices of family disturbance and
parental deviance were associated with psychiatric disorder in
the children (Rutter, 1973; Rutter et al., 1975b). In both
areas severe marital discord (see Quinton, Rutter and Rowlands,
1976) was considerably commoner in the families of children with
psychiatric disorder (Fig. 1), meaning that unhappy, disruptive,
quarrelsome homes were associated with child psychiatric disorder. Probably for the same reason, a "broken home" (that is a
home in which the child is not living with his two natural parents) was also associated with psychiatric disorder in London.
It was not associated with psychiatric disorder in the Isle of
Wight to the same extent, but this was explicable in terms of
the very different circumstances associated with broken homes
in the two areas (Rutter et al., 1975b). The proportion of children admitted "into care" and placed in Children's Homes or with
foster families is another index of family disturbance. Children admitted to short-term, as well as long-term, care frequently

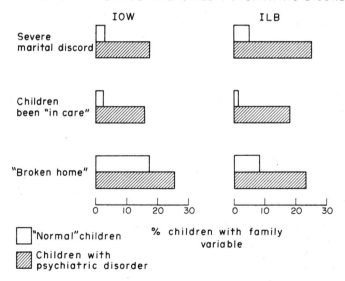

FAMILY DISTURBANCE AND CHILD PSYCHIATRIC DISORDER

Fig. 1

98   M. Rutter

come from and return to disturbed families (Schaffer and Schaffer, 1968; Wolkind and Rutter, 1973). Among the normal children in both areas only about 2% had been admitted into care
for as long as one continuous week, but among those with psychiatric disorder the proportion was 16-19%. Thus, as in other
studies (Rutter, 1971), family discord and disturbance was found
to be strongly associated with psychiatric disorder in the children.

Mental disorder in the mother, as assessed from a systematic
interview with her was associated with psychiatric problems in
the Isle of Wight children (Fig. 2). Half of the mothers of
children with psychiatric disorder has some form of psychiatric
condition themselves, compared with a rate of only 10% in the
mothers of normal children. Most of the maternal disorders consisted of mild chronic or recurrent depressive or neurotic conditions. The same association of disorder between mother and
child was not found in London probably because of the very high
rate of disorder in the mothers of the normal children and because in London women were less often associated with family
relationship difficulties (Rutter and Quinton, 1977). In both
populations the mean score on a health questionnaire which
tapped neurotic and psychosomatic symptoms was significantly
higher for the mothers of children with psychiatric problems.

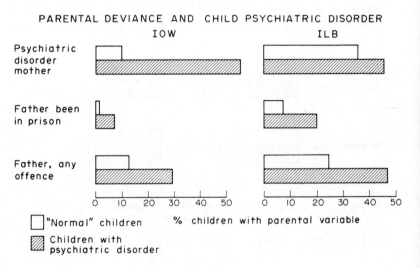

Fig. 2

Few of the fathers in both normal groups had been in prison and the rate in the fathers of the children with disorder was three times as high. Considering any offences against the law, again the rate was twice as high in the fathers of children with psychiatric disorder. The associations found between parental illness and deviance of various sorts and child psychiatric disorder is in keeping with other research findings (Rutter, 1966). Other factors associated with child psychiatric disorder included large family size, overcrowding and low social status.

TABLE 1 Family Adversity Index

---

1. Father : Unskilled/semiskilled job
2. Overcrowding or large family size
3. Marital discord and/or broken home
4. Mother : depression/neurosis
   (questionnaire score/interview rating)
5. Child ever "in care"
6. Father : Any offence against law

In order to look in more detail at the ways in which these family influences operated, they were combined in the form of a "family adversity index" (Rutter and Quinton, 1977). Six variables found to be associated with problems in the child were each given a score of "1" if present, so that each child had a score on the index which was in the range 0 to 6. As followed from the findings already discussed, children with high scores on the index were much more likely to have a psychiatric condition that those with very low scores. But something else which was not expected also emerged from the analysis.

Children with only one chronic family stress had no increase in psychiatric risk over the children without any of the six family stresses. At first we thought that this might be an artefact stemming from which factors occurred in isolation. However, close examination of the data showed that this was not the case. No chronic family stress was significantly associated with problems in the children if the stress occurred completely on its own. But if two or more stresses were present together, the psychiatric risk went up several fold far beyond what would be expected on the basis of a simple summation of risks. In short, there was a true interaction between stresses, which markedly inflated the psychiatric risk.

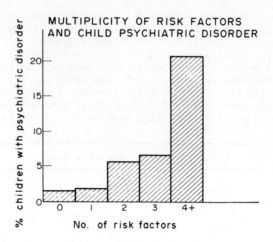

Fig. 3

More needs to be said about family influences but first it is
necessary to consider area differences.

AREA DIFFERENCES

Various studies have suggested major differences in rates of
psychiatric disorder and of delinquency between different geographical areas (see Rutter and Madge, 1976), but most studies
are open to the objection that they rely on administrative
statistics or that the methods of study used in the different
areas were not the same. We set out to investigate area differences with respect to psychiatric disorder in 10-year-old children by comparing the Isle of Wight with an inner London borough
(Rutter et al., 1975a and b). The same research strategy, the
same standardized methods and the same team of investigators
were used in both areas in order to eliminate artefactual differences in estimating prevalence of psychiatric disorder in
the two populations. As a further precaution we used a number
of different measures of psychiatric disorder.

The results were much the same however psychiatric disorder or
behavioural deviance was assessed; the rate was twice as high
in inner London as on the Isle of Wight (Fig. 4). This was so
for both boys and girls and for both emotional and conduct dis-

CHILD PSYCHIATRIC DISORDER/DEVIANCE
IN ISLE OF WIGHT (IOW) and LONDON (ILB)

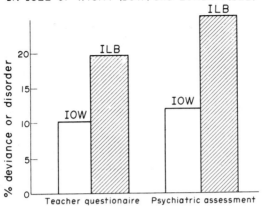

Fig. 4

orders. Furthermore, a series of methodological checks confirmed that the measures meant the same thing in the two areas and
that the area difference in psychiatric prevalence was valid.

The next question was: why are psychiatric disorders so much
more common in London? To answer that question we must utilize
the family adversity index which has already been mentioned. A
comparison of index scores in the two areas showed that three
times as many children in London were in families with at least
two stress factors. Could this explain the difference between
the two areas in rates of psychiatric disorder?

Table 2 shows that to a very large extent it does. When like
families in the two areas are compared there is no longer any
substantial difference in psychiatric rate between London and
the Isle of Wight. Thus, in both areas about a quarter of the
children living in families with a high family adversity score
showed psychiatric disorder. Similarly, in both areas among
those in more favoured family circumstances only about 10-15%
did so. In other words the difference in the prevalence of
child psychiatric disorder is almost entirely explicable in
terms of the much greater frequency of family adversity in the
two areas. The difference is completely eliminated if the area
difference in school adversity (see below) is also taken into
account.

TABLE 2
Child Psychiatric Disorder in London (ILB)
and Isle of Wight (IOW)
According to Family Adversity Index

	Family Adversity			
	Low score		High score	
	% with disorder	(Total N)	% with disorder	(Total N)
London	15.2%	(46)	30.0%	(50)
Isle of Wight	9.9%	(81)	25.0%	(20)

Of course, this finding immediately raises the issue of why family stress and adversity is so much more common in the metropolis. The answers to that question are still being sought but the findings already indicate that the explanation for the high rate of mental disorder in parents is rather different from that for the high rate in the children (Rutter and Quinton, 1977). For some reason the stresses of inner city life impinge particularly strongly on working class women (see also Brown et al., 1975). It is not just a question of low social status, as working class women on the Isle of Wight do not have an increased rate of psychiatric disorder. Why this should be so is not yet clear but in any case a consideration of the roots of family adversity take us beyond the theme of this paper.

SCHOOL VARIATION

Quite apart from area differences in rates of psychiatric disorder we found a marked variation between schools in the extent of behavioural deviance. Thus, in the study of inner London 10-year-olds, the proportion of children with deviant scores on the behavioural questionnaire completed by teachers was very much greater in some schools than others. Moreover, this behavioural variation between schools was systematically related to the characteristics of schools. For example, behavioural deviance was significantly more frequent in schools with high rates of teacher turnover or of pupil turnover (Fig. 5). In the same way as for family variables, the school characteristics associated with behavioural deviance were combined into a "school adversity index", the items of which are shown in Table 3.

SCHOOL CHARACTERISTICS AND CHILD DEVIANCE (ILB)

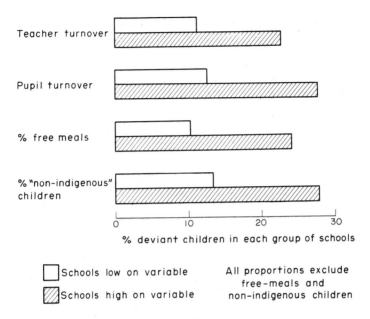

Fig. 5

TABLE 3   School Adversity Score

---

1. High proportion free school meals children
2. High proportion children of immigrants
3. High teacher turnover
4   High pupil turnover
5. High absenteeism
6. Low pupil : teacher ratio

TABLE 4
Behavioural Deviance in London
According to Family and School Adversity

| | | School Adversity | | | |
| | | Low | | High | |
		% deviant	Total N	% deviant	Total N
Family adversity	Low	0.0%	(21)	20.0%	(25)
	High	7.7%	(13)	27.0%	(37)

As follows from the way the index was derived, children attending schools with high scores on the index were much more likely
to be behaviourally deviant. The findings (see Table 4) also
show that, to some extent, well functioning schools can exert a
protective effect on children from disadvantaged or stressed
homes.

Of course, it is necessary to question whether the findings
could not be explained simply in terms of selective intake;
that is that some schools admit more "difficult" children than
do others. This possibility was difficult to exclude in the
case of primary school variation. We were able to show that the
school variation was not accounted for by the kinds of families
from which the children came (see Table 4). Furthermore,
schools characterized by, for example, a high proportion of
children eligible for free school meals (an index of relative
poverty) still had a high rate of behavioural deviance when the
analysis was confined to children in the school who were not
eligible for free meals. The circumstantial evidence suggested
that schools influenced children's behaviour but we could not
entirely rule out selective factors.

On the other hand, we could rule out selective factors in the
case of secondary schools if we followed the same group of children after transfer and into their new schools. Because we had
measures of the children's behaviour before transfer we could
partial out any biases in selective intake when examining variations between secondary schools. This is what we did. The
same London 10-year-olds were re-assessed at age 14 years in
their third year of secondary school.

It was necessary to take account of one further source of bias.

Because our main measure was a teacher questionnaire it was
possible that the school variation was a function of how teachers
perceived children or of how they completed questionnaires rather
than of how the children behaved. To examine this possibility
we took a number of other measures which were independent of
teacher judgement. These included rates of delinquency, of absenteeism and of reading difficulties (the children completed
group tests of reading and non-verbal intelligence).

As with primary schools, there were large differences between
secondary schools on all counts; questionnaire scores, delinquency rates, absenteeism and reading standards. However, we
also found a substantial bias in selection to the schools
(Rutter, 1977c) and this had to be taken into account statistically. We used both regression equations and standardization
procedures to partial out initial differences in the children's
behaviour and attainments prior to secondary transfer. The results were very closely similar with both methods (Rutter, 1977c).
Large differences between schools remained even after the appropriate statistical adjustments had been made in order to take
account of intake differences.

This is illustrated in Table 5 which shows the comparison between two schools with a rather similar intake of behaviourally
deviant children (Rutter, 1977c). A statistical regression technique (based on the correlation in the school population as a
whole between the question scores prior to transfer and in the
third year of secondary school) was used to take account of the
small intake difference and to predict the mean behavioural
questionnaire score expected if the school was exactly average
for the total group of schools. As Table 5 shows, both schools
could be expected to have a roughly similar questionnaire score.
In fact, one school had a much higher score than expected and
one had a far lower — the difference between them in this respect, if translated into numbers of deviant children, amounted
to a four fold difference in rate of deviance. Other analyses
showed that similar differences applied to delinquency rates,
absenteeism and (to a lesser extent) reading difficulties. The
variation was not just a matter of teacher perceptions.

It seemed clear that the children's behaviour had changed for
the better or worse according to which school they attended.
The next question is which aspect or feature of school life is
most important in this connection? What are the characteristics
of schools which have a beneficial effect on children's behavioural development? A detailed study of 12 schools is now in
progress in an attempt to answer that question.

TABLE 5 Regression Findings for Behavior Scale

| | Behavior scale age 10 years | | Predicted score at 14 years | | Actual score at 14 years | | Mean difference |
	Mean	S.D.	Mean	S.D.	Mean	S.D.	
School A Boys (n = 65)	6.59	6.67	4.62	1.20	2.59	4.15	-2.03
School B Boys (n = 50)	7.06	8.12	4.70	1.46	9.78	7.98	+5.08

AMELIORATING FACTORS

The last issue to be considered is the matter of ameliorating
factors. It is striking from all research findings that even
in the very worst situations some children develop well in spite
of all the stresses and disadvantages they experience. Why?
What is it that enables them to surmount the hazards they face?
This question has been a main focus in our recent work. Although
only a few findings are available so far, there are a number of
important leads (Rutter, 1977b). Some of these are relevant in
relation to the topic of this paper. .

Multiplicity of Stresses

First, as already discussed, there is the importance of multi-
plicity of stresses. If chronic family stresses are truly single,
there is little psychiatric risk. The problems for the child
occur when several stresses or disadvantages occur together.

Compensating Good Circumstances Outside the Home

Second, it is evident that good experiences at school can help
children even when they face difficulties and disadvantages at
home. We do not know whether a similar protective effect can
stem from other experiences outside the family — such as with
friends or in the community.

Temperamental Features

Third, research findings indicate that children's temperamental
characteristics play a major role in determining their vulnerability to psychiatric disorder (Graham, Rutter and George, 1973).
These were investigated in 3-7-year-old children in the study
of adult psychiatric patients' families (Rutter, 1971). Children who showed the features of low regularity, low malleability,
negative mood and low fastidiousness were the ones most at psychiatric risk. Children who had at least two of these adverse
temperamental features were three times as likely as other children to develop disorders during the next four years (Exact
test; $p = 0.027$). Figure 6 indicates one of the reasons why
this happens. Children subjected to frequent parental criticism
also had a much increased psychiatric risk. However, children
with adverse temperamental characteristics were twice as likely

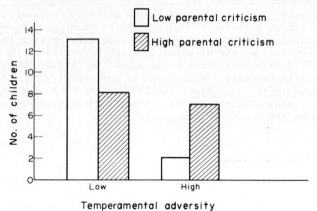

Fig. 6

as other children to be the target of parental criticism (Exact test; p = 0.054). When parents are depressed they do not "take it out" on all their children to the same extent. The child with "difficult" personality features tends to be the butt or scapegoat. Conversely, the easy, adaptable child tends to be protected even in a stressful home environment simply because much of the hostility and discord is focussed on other members of the family.

Heredity

Fourthly, studies of adopted or fostered children of adult criminals suggest that genetically vulnerable children are the ones most likely to succumb to environmental stresses (Hutchings and Mednick, 1974; Crowe, 1974). In other words, there is an important genetic-environmental interaction in which the one variable potentiates the effect of the other. Our own data do not enable a clear differentiation between genetic and environmental influences. However, the finding that the ill-effects of marital discord on the children are most marked in families in which one or both parents has a life-long personality disorder is suggestive of the same kind of interaction.

Good Relationships within the Home

Fifthly, it is necessary to consider modifying factors within
the home. As already noted, children are particularly likely
to develop conduct disorders when they are brought up in a discordant, quarrelsome, unhappy home. However, even in homes
characterized by marked discord between the parents many of the
children did not develop conduct disorders. One of the factors
which seemed to protect children in such circumstances was a
warm, positive relationship with one parent (see Fig. 7). Children who had a good relationship with at least one parent were
less than a third as likely to develop conduct disorders as
children whose relationships with both parents were poor.
Whether good relationships outside the home (such as with friends,
neighbours or other kin) have a similar protective effect is
not known but certainly the possibility needs to be investigated.

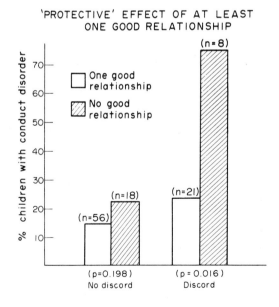

Fig. 7

Change in Family Circumstances

The last ameliorating factor to be considered is a change in
family circumstances for the better. In the study of patients
families we found that children, when young, who had experienced
stressful separations as a result of family discord or disorder
had a much increased risk of some form of conduct disorder
(Rutter, 1971). In order to examine the possible benefits of
improved family relationships we took this group of children,
all of whom had suffered stressful separations. Then, some
years later we compared those who were now in a harmonious family with those still living in a discordant home. The children
living in harmony had a rate of conduct disorder only a third
as high as the children who experienced continuing family discord. In short, behaviour and development is still modifiable
in middle and later childhood. Improved family circumstances
at that time brings benefits for the children. The damage done
by early stresses cannot be undone but it can be considerably
modified by experiences when older.

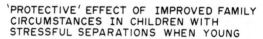

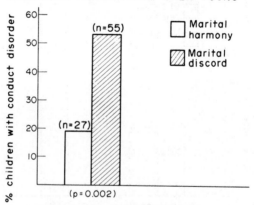

'PROTECTIVE' EFFECT OF IMPROVED FAMILY
CIRCUMSTANCES IN CHILDREN WITH
STRESSFUL SEPARATIONS WHEN YOUNG

Predominant family situation
during four year follow up period

Fig. 8

CONCLUSIONS

To summarize, family influences, area and community influences
and school influences all play a part in the genesis of conduct
disorders in childhood. The factors are multiple and tend to
interact to produce a complicated set of associations and relationships. Nevertheless, although much has still to be learned,
we are beginning to understand the processes and mechanisms involved.

Single chronic stresses are surprisingly unimportant if the
stresses really are isolated. The damage comes from multiple
stress and disadvantage, with different adversities interacting
and potentiating each other's influence. Genetic vulnerability
and environmental hazards also tend to interact in a way which
their power is increased. Nevertheless, in all these circumstances, there is immense individual variation and it is essen-
tial that we focus on the question of why many children do <u>not</u>
succumb to the perils they face. The reasons why they do not
are to be found not only in the characteristics of the individuals themselves, but also in the balance of good and bad influences they experience as they develop.

REFERENCES

Brown, G.W. and Rutter, M.L. (1966) The measurement of family
    activities and relationships: a methodological study,
    Human. Rel. 19, 241-263.

Brown, G.W., Bhrolchain, M.N. and Harris, T. (1975) Social
    class and psychiatric disturbance among women in an urban
    population, Sociology, 9, 225-254.

Crowe, R.R. (1974) An adoption study of antisocial personality,
    Arch. Gen. Psychiat. 31, 785-791.

Graham, P., Rutter, M. and George, S. (1973) Temperamental
    characteristics as predictors of behavior disorders in chil-
    dren, Amer. J. Othopsychiat. 43, 328-339.

Hutchings, B. and Mednick, S.A. (1974) Registered criminality
    in the adoptive and biological parents of registered male
    adoptees, in Mednick, S.A., Schulsinger, F., Higgins, J. &
    Bell, B. (eds.), Genetics, Environment and Psychopathology.
    Amsterdam, North Holland.

Quay, H.C. (1972) Patterns of aggression, withdrawal, and
    immaturity, in Quay, H.C. & Werry, J.S. (eds.), Psychopath-
    ological Disorders of Childhood. New York, Wiley.

Quinton, D., Rutter, M. and Rowlands, O. (1976) An evaluation
    of an interview assessment of marriage, Psychol. Med. 6,
    577-586.

Robins, L.N. (1966) Deviant Children Grown Up. Baltimore,
    Williams & Wilkins.

Rutter, M. (1966) Children of Sick Parents: An Environmental
    and Psychiatric Study. Institute of Psychiatry Maudsley
    Monographs No. 16. London, Oxford University Press.

Rutter, M. (1967) A children's behaviour questionnaire for
    completion by teachers: preliminary findings, J. Child
    Psychol. Psychiat. 8, 1-11.

Rutter, M. (1970) Sex differences in children's responses to
    family stress, in Anthony, E.J. & Koupernik, C. (eds.),
    The Child in His Family. New York, Wiley.

Rutter, M. (1971) Parent-child separation: psychological
    effects on the children, J. Child Psychol. Psychiatr. 12,
    233-260.

Rutter, M. (1973) Why are London children so disturbed?, Proc.
    Roy. Soc. Med. 66, 1221-1225.

Rutter, M. (ed.)(1977a) The Child, His Family and the Community.
    London, Wiley (in preparation).

Rutter, M. (1977b) Early sources of security and competence,
    in Bruner, J.S. and Garton, A. (eds.), Human Growth and
    Development. London, Oxford University Press.

Rutter, M. (1977c) Prospective studies to investigate behavioral
    change, in Strauss, J.S., Babigian, H.M. and Roff. M. (eds.),
    Methods of Longitudinal Research in Psychopathology. New
    York, Plenum (in press).

Rutter, M. and Brown, G.W. (1966) The reliability and validity
    of measures of family life and relationships in families
    containing a psychiatric patient, Soc. Psychiat. 1, 38-53.

Rutter, M. and Madge, N. (1976) Cycles of Disadvantage. London, Heinemann Educational.

Rutter, M. and Quinton, D. (1977) Psychiatric disorder — ecological factors and concepts of causation, in McGurk, H. (ed.), Ecological Factors in Human Development. Amsterdam, North Holland.

Rutter, M., Quinton, D. and Yule, B. (1977) Family Pathology and Disorder in Children. London, Wiley (in preparation).

Rutter, M., Tizard, J. and Whitmore, K. (eds.) (1970) Education, Health and Behaviour. London, Longmans Green.

Rutter, M., Cox, A., Tupling, C., Berger, M. and Yule, W. (1975a) Attainment and adjustment in two geographical areas: I. The prevalence of psychiatric disorder, Brit. J. Psychiat. 126, 493-509.

Rutter, M., Yule, B., Quinton, D., Rowlands, O., Yule, W., Berger, M. (1975b) Attainment and adjustment in two geographical areas: III. Some factors accounting for area differences, Brit. J. Psychiat. 126, 520-533.

Schaffer, H. and Schaffer, E.B. (1968) Child Care and the Family, Occasional Papers on Social Administration No. 25. London, Bell.

West, D.J. (1967) The Young Offender. London, Penguin Books.

Wolkind, S. and Rutter, M. (1973) Children who have been "in care": an epidemiological study, J. Child Psychol. Psychiat. 14, 95-105.

Yule, B. and Rutter, M. (1977) Unpublished data.

BEHAVIOURAL TREATMENT OF CHILDREN AND ADOLESCENTS WITH CONDUCT DISORDERS

W. Yule

INTRODUCTION

Conduct disorders in children and adolescents present one of
the major therapeutic challenges to professionals of all disciplines. It has long been recognized that the prognosis for
children with conduct disorders is poor (Robins, 1966), and
equally it has been widely recognized that traditional forms
of treatment are conspicuously less successful with conduct-
disordered children. Against this gloomy background, any form
of treatment which shows promise in helping children with conduct disorders is to be welcomed, but such a welcome need not
be uncritical.

The past 15 years has seen a dramatic increase in the number
of studies applying behavioural treatment to alleviating both
behavioural and emotional problems in child patients. These
techniques and their applications are described elsewhere
(Yule, 1976, 1977a). The present paper concentrates on their
application to the treatment of conduct disorders. Such applications are conceptually related to social-learning theory
formulations of anti-social behaviour in general, and aggressive behaviour in particular. Therefore, the paper begins by
outlining some of the findings of research stemming from social-
learning theory which has particular relevance to therapeutic
intervention.

This paper will then describe two major programmes of treatment:

(1) That of Dr. G.R. Patterson and his colleagues at the
    Oregon Research Institute. These investigators have
    developed an important therapeutic approach to help the
    families of aggressive boys.

(2) The second programme is that of Dr. M. Wolf and his col-
    leagues at the University of Kansas. They have developed
    a family-style token-economy approach to treating young
    delinquent boys.

In both sections, the work of other investigators will be
briefly described. Finally, the paper will consider some of the
methodological problems raised by these studies. In particular,
it will address the question of how such techniques can be used
in other settings and other cultures. Clearly, if it is accepted that behavioural techniques make a significant contribution
to the treatment of conduct disorders, it is important to know
how to replicate the treatments in other countries.

TREATMENT IMPLICATIONS FROM SOCIAL LEARNING THEORY

What is Social Learning Theory?

Social learning theory is concerned with explaining the development of behaviour in inter-personal, social settings. Many
would agree with Patterson (1969) when he says that "The term
social learning ... refers to the loosely organized body of literature dealing with the changes in learning, or performance,
which occur as a function of contingencies which characterize
social interaction." However, social learning theorists are
concerned with factors in addition to contingency management,
and broader formulations have been proposed by Bandura and his
colleagues (Bandura and Walters, 1963). For example, Ross (1974)
comments that "The behavioral orientation that guided my writing
places a great deal of emphasis on the all-important role of the
social environment in shaping and maintaining human behavior,
but it also makes room for such concepts as self-control, self-
observation, observational learning and cognitive mediations as
well as for a limited number of operationally defined constructs
such as anxiety and anger."

Thus, one of the cardinal features of social learning theory is
its conceptualization of psychological problems as either the
presence of maladaptive behaviours which have been learned or
as the absence of adaptive behaviours which have not yet been
learned. A second feature which follows from this formulation
is that the mechanisms involved in the acquisition and maintenance of deviant behaviour are the same as those involved in the
acquisition and maintenance of socially acceptable behaviour.
Thus, social learning theorists emphasize the importance of
normal mechanisms of learning for the understanding of the aetiology of disorders of behaviour and their maintenance.

A third feature of social learning theory is its emphasis on the
distinction between factors involved in the acquisition of a

behaviour problem and factors involved in its maintenance.
Irrespective of the origins of the problem, deviant behaviour
can often develop vicariously and be maintained by different
factors. It follows from this that the therapist focuses on the
here-and-now behaviour of the patient and the social environment
in which such behaviour is presenting. The treatment formulation may be a-historical, but it is certainly not a-contextual.
Treatment consists largely of identifying relevant features of
the social environment, manipulating them carefully, and evaluating the effects of such manipulation.

The Social Learning Theory View of Aggressive Behaviour

Bandura (1973), Berkowitz (1973) and Ross (1974) all provide important reviews of social learning theory approaches to the control of aggression. Readers are referred to these for more detailed consideration of the points discussed below, and for the
empirical underpinnings of much of what follows in this section.

The first point such social learning theorists make is that it
makes little sense to consider aggression as a trait. Instead,
the focus is on aggressive behaviour which must be considered
within the social context that it occurs. For example, if one
child hits another child with a hammer and causes injury, most
people would label the first child's behaviour as aggressive.
However, when one adult in a green uniform fires a gun at another adult in a red uniform in a situation where territory and
natural resources are under dispute, it is much more difficult
to get agreement on whether the act is aggressive. As Bandura
(1973) puts it, " ... aggression is characterized as injurious
and destructive behaviour that is socially defined as aggressive
on the basis of a variety of factors, some of which reside in
the evaluator rather than in the performer."

A second point made by such theorists is that what characterizes
much aggressive behaviour is the high magnitude of that behaviour. Pushing and shoving are common features of young children's behaviour at school. The child who pushes hard and pushes
frequently is the child who is likely to be labelled as aggressive.

A third point made particularly by Patterson, Littman and Bricker
(1967) in their monograph on Assertive Behaviour in Children is
that "Assertive behaviors are coercive in the sense that they
demand (force) a reaction from the environment, and very often,

the consequences are reinforcing ... the social environment is
so organized or programmed as to support the maintenance and
acquisition of a wide spectrum of assertive behaviors as a regular feature of the socialization process for the normal child.
Consequently the rare, high amplitude event "aggression" is a
reasonable outcome of certain specialized training procedures
that place many additional classes of behavior at high strength."

Most assertive behaviours in nursery school settings are of very
short duration and are of such amplitude that they go unnoticed
by the casual observer. The average pre-school quarrel lasts
between 15 and 36 seconds (Dawe, 1934), but when such brief,
low-amplitude assertive behaviour does occur, it is very likely
to be reinforced. In particular, Patterson, Littman and Bricker
(1967) draw attention to the reinforcing behaviour of the victim.
In 80% of incidents of assertive behaviour, the aggressor was
reinforced by the victims who yielded, gave up the object demanded, withdrew and so on. However, when the victim occasionally
retaliated, he was likely to be reinforced for his assertive
behaviour (on 69% of the occasions).

Thus, social learning theorists draw attention to the importance
of the peer group as well as the parent in shaping up aggressive
behaviour. In their nursery school study, Patterson, Littman
and Bricker (1967) showed that the school setting is such that
assertive behaviour is reinforced by both teachers and peers.
It was found that most children who entered as fairly passive
beings soon learned to be assertive. Thus, from a social learning viewpoint, the problem is not so much to account for why
children become assertive and aggressive, but rather to account
for why more children do not become assertive. In other words,
there is a shift of focus on to the mechanisms whereby most
children learn to inhibit aggressive behaviour.

A fifth group of points to emerge from more recent social learning analyses of aggressive and anti-social behaviour within
family settings relates to the findings of Patterson and his
colleagues (see Patterson and Reid, 1970) that the mechanisms
whereby assertive or coercive behaviour is reinforced are somewhat different from the mechanisms operating in classrooms.
Whereas pro-social behaviours are usually learned under a system
of positive reinforcement, it appears that many deviant behaviours are learned under a system of negative reinforcement
(Patterson and Cobb, 1971). What happens is that the assertive
or coercive behaviour of the child demands a response from the
parent. All too often, this response is negative. The child

continues with his whining or demanding or whatever, and the
parent likewise escalates his or her refusal to give in. Eventually, after both parent and child have escalated their by-now-
unpleasant behaviour, one party gives in. The effect of the
parent's intermittent capitulation is to provide an escape from
an unpleasant situation and thereby increase the likelihood that
the child will behave in the demanding, assertive manner in the
future.

Studies of mother-child interaction show that mothers of young
children referred to clinics on account of behavioural disturbance, issue more frequent commands and use more criticism than
do mothers of non-clinic children (Forehand et al., 1975). However, when parents of normal children want their children to
misbehave, they too increase the number of commands they give
the children (Johnson and Lobitz, 1974). Thus, the behaviour
of parents is clearly important in both initiating the chain of
coercive behaviours by issuing too many commands, and in maintaining it by negative reinforcement.

Patterson, and others, draw attention to the widespread finding
in many studies that parents of aggressive, anti-social children
often behave inconsistently towards their children, particularly
where discipline is concerned. Punishment can be erratic;
assertiveness is often openly encouraged. Recent findings
(Patterson, 1965; Patterson, Cobb and Ray, 1973) suggest that
children in such homes become indifferent to the normal range
of social reinforcers normally given by parents to their children. The implication of such findings is that reinforcement
is not enough and consistency is not enough. Such children have
to relearn that parental attention and parental pleasure in
achievement is reinforcing. How this is attempted will be described later.

Thus, different mechanisms of social learning may operate in
different settings. The implication of this is that changing
behaviour in one setting involving alterations in one set of
mechanisms will not necessarily generalize to another setting.
Improvement in behaviour at home may not automatically generalize to behaviour at school. Both settings will have to be worked
in.

Sixthly, in keeping with the view that the same psychological
mechanisms underlie the development of both normal and deviant
behaviour, the treatment principles and practices involved in
helping children with conduct disorders are basically the same

as those involved in all behavioural treatment. These are described in more detail elsewhere (Yule, 1976, 1977a). However,
the relative emphasis on treatment procedures differs.

From what has been said earlier, it is clear that the usual techniques of positive shaping using positive, social reinforcement
has an important but, at least in early stages, a limited role.
Whilst it is important to teach parents and teachers the value
of positive reinforcement techniques, until the conduct disorders are seen to be under some sort of control, it is difficult
for parents to see the relevance of such changes in their own
behaviour.

Even so, it is vital that such positive shaping techniques are
learned since one of the most powerful ways of reducing undesirable behaviour is to increase an incompatible set of desirable
behaviours. Children presenting with conduct problems often
don't know how to behave any differently. Social learning therapists say "Teach them"! Thus, a necessary part of the behaviour
therapists' functional analysis of a conduct problem is to identify alternative, competing, pro-social behaviours already in
the child's repertoire, and consider how these might be strengthened. Bandura (1969, 1973) lays great emphasis on the importance of modelling in respect of learning such new behaviour
patterns.

As far as learning to inhibit anti-social behaviour is concerned,
there are two main lines of investigation of relevance. The
first concerns the stimulus settings which cue or set-off anti-
social episodes. Aggression is more likely to occur if imple-
ments associated with aggression are present (Berkowitz, 1973).
Absconding is more likely to occur in dark nights (Clarke and
Martin, 1971). By identifying any discriminant stimuli which
are often present during anti-social incidents, the therapist
can alter the environment and so avoid the problem. This is
obviously a useful thing to do, but can hardly be seen as an
ideal solution.

The second line of investigation into self-control concerns the
normal developmental sequence of learning social inhibitions.
Most people are agreed that there is a need for external controls coming from adults before the child can learn self-control.
There is increasing interest from cognitive psychologists in
the regulatory functions of language on behaviour. Getting
children to rehearse aloud the rationalization for their actions,
and, probably more importantly, labelling what they are doing,

is seen as potentially effective in inhibiting unacceptable
behaviour.

A seventh group of points to come from contemporary social learning theory is related to the reinstatement of punishment as a
powerful regulator of children's undesirable activities (Cheyne,
1972). Punishment is susceptible to the same detailed analysis
as is reinforcement, and not surprisingly it is discovered that
the timing, severity, consistency and identification of alternative behaviours are all important dimensions which need consideration (Walters, Cheyne and Banks, 1972).

No one is advocating the use of unnecessarily harsh punishment.
"Time-out from positive reinforcement" as part of a planned
treatment programme has been well described by a number of authors (Patterson and Gullion, 1968; Clark et al., 1973; MacDonough and Forehand, 1973; Sachs, 1973). "Time-out" is most
effective when it is of short duration - up to 5 or 10 minutes.
Any longer, and effectively the child is being prevented from
learning a more appropriate way of dealing with the difficult
situation. As with all techniques, there are wide individual
differences in children's responses (Hops and Walters, 1963),
and only careful record keeping will indicate whether the technique is useful in any individual case.

Time out from positive reinforcement can be seen as a particular
application of extinction procedures. In theory, if a behaviour
has been maintained at a high rate by (usually intermittent)
reinforcement, then, when that reinforcement is no longer made
available, the behaviour will weaken and eventually extinguish.
This procedure is time consuming, and not advisable when aggressive behaviours are the subject of concern. Whilst extinction
can work with aggressive behaviour (Brown and Elliott, 1965),
mostly parents and teachers will not risk the possibility of
another child being hurt while the treatment is taking effect.

Berkowitz (1973) makes the telling point that there is always
the danger that when an adult studiously ignores inappropriate
behaviour, the child may interpret this as tacit approval of his
actions. As noted earlier, this danger can be avoided by explaining to the child what is being ignored and why.

In summary, social learning theory has many practical implications for adults trying to help children overcome conduct problems. Behavioural treatment focuses on the here-and-now situation, and tries to understand the problems within the framework

of maladaptive learning in an interpersonal-social setting.
High intensity problems such as aggression are seen as but a
subset of more general assertive behaviours which are compara-
tively easier to bring under control.

Whilst techniques of positive reinforcement of pro-social behaviour play an important role in behavioural treatment, they are
not sufficient to initiate the reduction of many anti-social
behaviours. These have often been learned and maintained in a
coercive system where negative reinforcement has been applied
inconsistently. Such experiences reduce the potency of ordinary social reinforcers. Hence, there is an emphasis on external
controls and the use of systematic, consistent, but relatively
mild punishment in the early stages of treatment. Punishment
is never used in isolation. Behavioural techniques emphasize
the important of training up incompatible, socially desirable
behaviours.

In carrying out a functional analysis of the problem (Yule, 1977b),
the therapist gets a good, objective description of the problem
in observable terms. He will try to get reliable data counts to
establish the frequency of the problem and the circumstances in
which it occurs. He will enquire into other behaviours present
in the child's repertoire which could be strengthened so as to
replace the undesired behaviour. He will consider what reinforcers and what punishers are available to the adults who will
actually treat the child.

Behavioural treatments, then, are a sophisticated set of techniques having a close relationship to social learning theory.
They are empirically based, and can be applied flexibly and sen-
sitively to a wide range of conduct problems. The emphasis on
data collection and evaluation of treatment outcome quickly
tells the therapist if and when a particular course of treatment
requires readjustment. In the sections which follow, two such
flexible and successful programmes will be described which il-
lustrate the behavioural approach to treating conduct disorders.

BEHAVIOURAL TREATMENT WITH FAMILIES AND INDIVIDUALS IN NON-INSTITUTIONAL SETTINGS (the work of G.R. Patterson and his colleagues)

About ten years ago, Dr. Patterson and his colleagues at the
Oregon Research Institute began exploring the application of
behavioural techniques to the treatment of aggressive behaviour.

Spurred on by the success of their initial case studies, they rapidly developed a "treatment package" which involves primarily training the parents of the aggressive children. The development and details of this treatment approach are described in a number of publications (Patterson, Cobb and Ray, 1973; Patterson and Reid, 1973; Patterson, 1974a).

Briefly, the procedure is as follows. Boys are referred from some community agency because of some type of conduct problem. Consecutive referrals are offered treatment, which consists of a sequence of three or four stages.

Firstly, both parents have to read a semi-programmed text explaining the principles of behaviour modification. The specially written texts are Living With Children (Patterson and Gullion, 1968) and Families: Applications of Social Learning Theory to Family Life (Patterson, 1971). Only when one of these had been read and parents showed evidence of understanding them by passing a multiple-choice test were they allowed to go on to the second stage.

The second stage involved project staff teaching the parents to pinpoint behaviours of concern and to collect appropriate data on them. Once they had successfully collected sufficient data they moved on to stage three.

The third stage involved joining a small parent training group containing 3 or 4 sets of parents. These groups met weekly and modelling and role-playing procedures were used to teach appropriate techniques. The programme which parents devized was monitored and any alterations necessary were worked out in collaboration with the professionals. Discussion of problems was usually made contingent on the presentation of data.

Fourthly, if little or no change was apparent after 10 to 12 weeks home visits were arranged and more intensive analyses of problems were undertaken.

On average, each treatment programme lasted about 3 to 4 months. Early on in the programme of research, it was discovered that gains made at home did not generalize to the schools. A separate, parallel treatment package was developed for use in school settings (Patterson, Cobb and Ray, 1972).

The results of this approach are both promising and impressive. The research group has paid a great deal of attention to methodology and to the development of reliable instruments to measure change. In particular, they have developed a complex observation procedure whereby trained observers visit the homes and gather direct data on family interactions. Outcomes are reported in terms of their observational data, as well as in terms of the data gathered by parents.

The main study has been reported in detail (Patterson, 1974a, 1974b, 1974c). From January 1968 to June 1972, 35 boys with recognized conduct disorders were referred for treatment. Families containing severely retarded, acutely psychotic or severely brain damaged members were excluded from the trial, leaving 27 families who entered treatment and remained in treatment for at least four weeks. The majority of families were from lower socio-economic levels, and fathers were absent in eight instances.

Follow-up data were obtained monthly for the first six months after termination of treatment, and thereafter every two months until 12 months after termination.

Training the families took an average of 31.5 hours of professional time. Later, "booster" treatment during follow-up occupied an average of a further 1.9 hours of professional time.

Three types of criterion measures were gathered in the homes:

1) Targetted deviant child behaviours. Most parents chose to work on reducing the amount of non-compliance to requests shown by their sons. A further 13 behaviours (such as teasing, yelling, destructiveness) were pin-pointed by parents during treatment. From observational data, the rates of occurrence of each of these behaviours actually worked on were computed. From baseline level to termination there was, on average, a 60% reduction in the rates at which the undesirable behaviour occurred. In three out of four cases, reductions exceeded 30% from baseline levels. In only six cases did the rate of targetted behaviour get worse.

2) Total deviant scores. Rates of deviant behaviour over 14 problem areas observed during home visits were computed. Initially, the 27 boys showed significantly higher overall rates than did normal boys. By the end of intervention, the rate had dropped to just within the normal limit. During follow-up, there was initially a slight rise followed by a progressive fall in the rate of occurrence of deviant behaviours. At the one-year follow-up, the group of initially aggressive boys was indistinguishable from the normal boys on whom the observations had been piloted.

3) Parent daily report. As the study progressed, data gathering was improved. Data were obtained from 14 families and showed a significant drop in the level of reported problems during follow-up. About two-thirds of the families reported marked reductions in the problems for which they were originally referred.

On all three sets of criterion measures, statistical analysis showed that the changes were highly significant. Recently, Patterson (1975) has summarized the effects of his treatment programme as follows:

"... the emphasis was on buttressing both parental social reinforcers and punishment in the context of contractual arrangements between child, parent and school. The clinical findings show that indeed most parents could be taught to perform these skills. While no formal analysis has been done, it is the writer's (i.e. Patterson's) impression that for about a third of the families, it is sufficient to adopt the simplest possible strategy, e.g. teach the parent the specific skills for changing child behaviours. Another third of the families seem to require much more than this, including the teaching of negotiation skills, resolution of marital conflict and depression being the most common. Our attempts to develop such supplementary techniques are described in Patterson, Weiss and Hops (1975). If these problems are not dealt with, we believe the long-term follow-up will show the treatment to have been ineffective. The remaining one-third fail in spite of our best efforts."

There have been many other studies associated with this exciting programme. Wiltz and Patterson (1974) used a waiting list control group to test the effects of 5 weeks of parent training. The treatment group produced significant decreases in the observed rates of deviant child behaviour, whereas the rates in the waiting list controls remained steady.

Walter and Gilmore (1973) also used parents from the main study. Twelve consecutive referrals were placed in either the treatment programme or a placebo treatment group. The placebo group met an equal number of times, but had general discussions of their children's problems. The treatment group showed significant decreases in the rates of deviant behaviour, whereas the placebo-treatment group showed non-significant increases in rates of deviant behaviour.

Eyberg and Johnson (1974) used different observers and therapists, and worked with 15 younger aggressive boys. They too obtained

a significant reduction of targetted deviant child behaviours.
The reduction amounted to 40% over baseline levels. This con-
stitutes a satisfactory replication of the treatment package.

Although Eyberg's replication was independent of Patterson's
group, his therapists had been trained by people who had had the
good fortune to work with Patterson. Ferber, Keeley and Shemberg (1974) report an attempted replication with less favourable
outcome. Working well away from Oregon, and training themselves
on the basis of published information, they worked with seven
children. Some positive short term results were found in three
of the seven families, but at one-year follow-up all but one
family still reported serious problems. However, the follow-up
data were obtained by telephone and not by direct observation.
Thus on a number of counts, this study cannot be seen as an adequate attempt to replicate Patterson's approach. Nevertheless,
it warns of the dangers of diluting an established treatment
package.

One final study relating to Patterson's work is worth mentioning
in the context of the present paper. It emerges that boys who
are not only aggressive, but who also steal, are more difficult
to treat. Using as criterion of success in treatment a 33% reduction in the rate of deviant behaviour, Reid and Hendricks
(1973) looked more closely at the previously mentioned 27 families. They found that 6 of 14 stealers compared with 9 of 11 non-
stealers were classified as successes (data were missing on two
cases). It was found that the stealers exhibited less overall
deviant behaviour, and that they came from families which exhibited much lower rates of positive, friendly behaviours. Clearly,
the wealth of data gathered in studies such as these are inval-
uable in leading both to a better understanding of the dynamics
of families of aggressive children, and to effective methods for
treating the problems in the natural environment.

Other investigators have also worked with delinquents and their
families using behavioural interventions. One of the earliest
published studies was that by Tharp and Wetzel (1969) who used
non-professionals as therapists for young delinquents. Of 135
single case studies carried out, the targetted behaviours fell
to below 50% of baseline level in no fewer than 120 instances.
There were 77 children in this study — 26 had committed offences
prior to treatment and only 5 committed further offences in the
following 6 months.

Alexander and Parsons (1973) compared the use of short-term fam-

ily behavioural treatment (N = 46) with client-centred family
groups (N = 19), eclectic psychodynamic family treatment (N = 11)
and no-treatment control (N = 10). In the county in which they
worked, the general recidivism rate for delinquents was 51%.
In their study, the recidivism rates in the 6 to 18 months post-
treatment were respectively 26% (behavioural), 47% (client-centred), 73% (psychodynamic) and 50% (control). The authors concluded that a focus on families per se is not sufficient to modify family interaction patterns or to reduce rates of delinquency.
Behavioural methods offer something more, but just what that
something is has not yet been clearly defined.

Davidson and Seidman (1974) review studies of behaviour modification and delinquency which were published in the 13 years from
1960 to 1973. They remind us that there is a close relationship
between delinquency and educational disorders (Rutter and Yule,
1970). They note that significant educational gains can be made
by delinquents given behavioural help. Overall, the studies
show promising results, but there were sufficient methodological
problems noted to make the reviewers cautious about making pre-
mature claims of dramatic success.

There is no space within the present paper to deal with the very
large literature on behaviour modification in school settings.
It is clear from reading this literature that many of the problems tachers have successfully dealt with are conduct problems.
Those interest in following up work in this area are referred
to O'Leary and O'Leary (1972), Ward (1975), Thoreson (1973),
Sherman and Bushell (1975).

The overall impression given by this literature is that behaviour
modification techniques have gained a wide measure of acceptance
in a relatively short period of time. There is a great deal of
healthy research in progress, and the data-based nature of the
treatment approach pays handsome dividends in leading to a better
understanding of the nature of conduct disorders. Nowhere was
this more evident than in the research carried out by Patterson
and his colleagues.

BEHAVIOURAL TREATMENT IN RESIDENTIAL SETTINGS
(the Achievement Place Project)

The preceding section was largely concerned with studies which
aimed to help conduct disordered children in their own homes or
schools. However, as we know (Clarke and Cornish, 1976), many

such children are taken out of their homes, often out of their
communities, and cared for in residential settings - usually with
little observable benefit. As Cornish and Clarke (1975) argued,
there is a need for more effective treatment within residential
homes. This section will focus on one project which aims to do
this.

"Achievement Place is a community-based, family-style, behavior
modification, group home for six to eight delinquent or predelinquent youths from 12 through 15 years old" (Wolf, Phillips
and Fixsen, 1975). It is based in Lawrence, Kansas, and the
home is actually located in the community in which the youths
normally reside. Thus, even though they have been sent to
Achievement Place by the courts, they continue to attend their
normal schools and can visit their own homes regularly. Scep-
tics might add that they are therefore still in contact with the
peer group influences that got them into trouble in the first
place!

The philosophy of the Kansas group is that the boys do not suffer
from some internal psychopathology. Rather, they are seen as
lacking in appropriate social skills. "The goal of the behavioral treatment programme, therefore, is to establish through
reinforcement, modelling and instruction, the important behavioral competencies in social (including interpersonal relationship skills), academic, prevocational and self-care skills that
the youths have not acquired" (Wolf, Phillips and Fixsen, 1975).

The task of training the boys is entrusted to a couple who are
specially trained to act as houseparents. For good reasons,
they are called "teaching parents". They live in on the job,
24 hours a day, just like parents. Their job is to make full
use of every opportunity to teach appropriate skills to the boys
in their care. They are well trained in behaviour modification
techniques, and they have the responsibility for defining target behaviours, executing programmes, and keeping data in addition to running the house.

Since it is a family-style unit, there are no outside domestics.
All the boys co-operate in domestic chores. Besides keeping
costs down, this has the very desirable effect of teaching the
boys self-care skills that they would otherwise have no opportunity to learn.

There are four main aspects to the Achievement Place treatment
package:

(1) The motivation system. The whole house is run on very
sophisticated token economy lines. Boys earn points for achiev-
ing specified goals; they lose points for infractions of the
rules.

(2) The self-government system. At the evening meal, there is
a family discussion. Here, boys are helped to participate in
making the rules of the house. The teaching-parents retain
ultimate sanctions, but the boys quickly learn to take on a
great deal of responsibility for their own behaviour.

(3) The comprehensive behavioural skill training curriculum.
In keeping with their skills-training philosophy, wherever a
skill deficit is identified, then a suitable remedial programme
is worked out. For example, when boys were found to be defi-
cient in skills required in going for job interviews, remedial
training was successfully worked out in that area (Braukmann et
al., 1974). When a boy did not appear to know how to introduce
himself to strangers, a social skills training programme was
worked out. After participating in the programme, the boy would
greet the person, make good eye contact, smile and make appropriate conversation (Phillips et al., 1976, in press).

Another example of this approach involves one more area of typical skill deficit in delinquent teenagers - conflict between
parents and children. Often conflicts arise because neither
party has appropriate skills in negotiating solutions which involve making realistic compromises. Kifer et al. (1974) describe an active treatment approach which involves training both
parents and children to clarify the conflict situation; to list
the options open; to consider the consequences of each option;
and then to simulate a negotiation situation. This positive,
educational approach has clear application in many families seen
at psychiatric clinics.

(4) The relationship between youths and the teaching-parents.
This is clearly an important component in the whole treatment
package. It is important to note that the relationship is generally non-authoritarian and avowedly educational.

Achievement Place has been in existence for about nine years.
Recently, Wolf and his colleagues have described the outcome of
the first 41 boys to be admitted (Wolf, Phillips and Fixsen,
1975). Their average age was 13.8 years (range 10-16), 61%
were white, 29% black; two-thirds came from families with one
or neither parent at home; 53% of the families were on welfare;
their average IQ was 97 (range 73-113) and about two-thirds had

severe educational difficulties. All the boys had been placed
by the courts; 95% had previously had contact with probation or
psychology clinic services; 68% had been in jail; 43% had been
in previous residential care. In other words, this was a very
deprived group of boys who all had severe conduct disorders.

The treatment programme has been evaluated in a number of ways.
The harshest test is to look at the outcome in terms of later
institutionalization and reconviction. The first 18 boys placed
in Achievement Place were compared with 19 boys placed in a local
reformatory. In the two years following treatment, 3 of the
Achievement Place boys (22%) compared with 9 of the reformatory
boys (47%) were placed in other institutional care. Court contacts decreased among Achievement Place boys during the treatment, but increased among boys at the reformatory.

At the two-year follow-up, the average number of court contacts
of the Achievement Place boys was 1.7 and 55% of the boys were
still attending a school programme. By contrast, the boys in
the reformatory had an average of 1.5 court contacts and only
33% were enrolled in any educational programme (in the first
year after discharge). The differences in treatment procedures
necessitated the difference in length of follow-up between the
groups, but these findings on recidivism and school attendance
are encouraging. In addition, the preliminary data indicate
that the cost of treatment in Achievement Place was substantially
less than the cost of treatment in the institution.

One of the criticisms that is frequently levelled at any behavioural programme which uses tokens and tangible reinforcers is
that the children will become self-interested materialists.
Eitzen (1975) undertook an independent evaluation of changes in
attitudes of boys who had been in the Achievement Place programme. He found that "The greatest shifts in attitude were from
poor to good self-esteem and from externality to internality.
Not only were these changes more favourable over time, but they
were more dramatic - from much more negative than the comparison
group at the beginning to much more favourable than the comparison group at the end." (Eitzen, 1975). He further found no support for the idea that the boys became more scheming and Machia-
vellian.

Achievement Place is a carefully thought out, sophisticated and
comprehensive approach to the treatment of young delinquents.
The programme has been clearly described in a number of publications (Phillips, 1968; Phillips et al., 1972, 1973; Wolf,

Phillips and Fixsen, 1975), and reference will be found there
to the many other studies investigating the contribution of different components to the total treatment package. It is notable
that at the time of writing, there are at least 35 replication
homes in existence in America, and NIMH have sponsored an independent evaluation of their efficacy.

Braukmann and Fixsen (1976, in press) have recently reviewed
other behavioural approaches to the treatment of delinquents.
Many of the other programmes - such as that of Cohen and Filipczak (1971) - are carried out within closed institutions. This
makes the problem of obtaining generalization of effects much
more critical. Even so, Braukmann and Fixsen (1976) were im-
pressed by the variety both in the behaviours dealt with and the
techniques developed. They note that over the years there has
been a welcome shift in the focus of treatment from a concern to
suppress unwanted behaviour to a concern with increasing desirable behaviours. This latter trend calls into question the
appropriateness of the training of staff who have responsibility
for caring for delinquents.

In summary, the Achievement Place model demonstrates that behavioural techniques can be used flexibly and imaginatively within
a group home setting dealing with young delinquents. The boys
can remain largely in their usual community and by carefully
grading their return home, the improvements in social skills and
in self control appear to be more efficient than traditional
institutional treatments in preventing recidivism.

CURRENT PROBLEMS AND FUTURE DEVELOPMENTS

Within the confines of this paper, I have chosen to give lengthy
descriptions of two of the most interesting programmes of research into applying behavioural techniques to conduct disorders,
rather than attempt a statistical-style summary of all published
studies. In this way, I hope that I have illustrated how the
principles of treatment derived from social learning theory formulations can be used in real-life treatment situations. It is
clear that such programmes are very sophisticated and also very
flexible and sensitive to the needs of the individuals they are
trying to help.

Even so, there are a great many questions still to answer. It
is said that one hallmark of good research is that it ends up
with more unanswered questions than it started - but that the

questions have been clarified and are posed in a manner that
permits of rigorous investigation. This is true of much of the
behavioural research into conduct disorders.

From the programmes described earlier, it is clear that there
can be a close and fruitful relationship between pure and applied
research. Patterson's detailed home-observations of family
interaction patterns not only provide data relating to the efficacy of treatment, but they cast light on factors important in
the aetiology and maintenance of aggressive behaviour. Studies
such as those of Staats and Butterfield (1965) where delinquents
are taught to read may help to clarify the connection between
academic failure and conduct disorder. Already it is obvious
that a social learning analysis can go a long way towards understanding the development and maintenance of conduct disorders.

Sophisticated as they are, published studies still suffer from
a number of methodological problems. These are, of course, not
peculiar to studies of behaviour modification. For example,
there is widespread disagreement on the use of recidivism rates
as criterion measures for outcome. Leaving that to one side,
there are major problems in comparing outcomes across groups
when the rehabilitation policies of the different agencies may
mean that some children are longer back in their home community
than others. The early-released boys have greater opportunities
to commit further offences (Cornish and Clarke, 1975; Wolf,
Phillips and Fixsen, 1975). One way of overcoming the problem
of objections to a single criterion measure is, of course, to
use a number of different outcome measures. If all measures
show improvement in the same direction, then the incremental
validity lends weight to the interpretation of the findings
(Patterson, 1974b).

The problem of selecting appropriate comparison groups is always
present in real-life, field trials. Random allocation of boys
to treatments is one way of overcoming selection biases, and is,
in part, being undertaken currently at Achievement Place in
that since there are more than three applicants for every vac-
ancy, they select one at random and follow the others, wherever
they are sent (Wolf, Phillips and Fixsen, 1975).

As far as evaluating series is concerned, Patterson (1974a) makes
the following points: consecutive referrals should be accepted
and outcome reported relating to the total group; evaluation
data should be obtained by other than the therapist or the client;
follow-up data should be obtained to examine the persistence of

the effects; data should be gathered to examine the extent to
which any treatment effects generalize to other settings; and
evidence should be presented to demonstrate that the treated
group do better than untreated controls. Costly as this may
seem, without such data we will not be in a position to choose
effective treatments for conduct disorders on a rational basis.
Only a few studies approximate to this high level of evaluative
sophistication.

Patterson's list of requirements mentions a number of problem
areas which should be highlighted. Firstly, there is the problem of generalization. As the evidence mounts up, it becomes
clearer that children's behaviour is much more situation specific than was once believed. Whilst this is in accord with social
learning formulations of behaviour, it means that unless generalization of effects is planned for, it is unlikely to occur
spontaneously (Patterson and Brodsky, 1966). As was seen earlier, treatment often has to be carried out simultaneously in
the home and the school. Further, it implies that the trend to
treat in the natural environment rather than in the clinic will
have to be accelerated. The natural social environment includes
the child's parents and teachers, and more direct training of
these groups can be anticipated (Yule, 1975).

The second major, but related, problem is that of maintenance
of therapeutic change. Many more long-term follow-up studies
are needed. Whilst it is exciting to be able to produce short-
term changes, a more thorough understanding of the mechanisms
of maintenance is required. This has led to an increased interest in the area of "self-control" (Cautela, 1969; Thoresen and
Mahoney, 1974). Hopefully, further research into the cognitive
variables involved will increase the number of techniques for
ensuring the maintenance of behavioural change.

Another whole area of questions concern what is being called
the "process studies" in this area. The large programmes described are complex treatment packages. Ultimately, what is
needed is a better understanding of the separate contributions
of the constituent components. This is provided by smaller
scale experimental studies, including single-case studies. It
has become clear that there is a complex interaction between
the behaviour to be changed, the measure of outcome taken, and
the appropriate single-case research design required to demonstrate change (Matthews, 1975; Yule and Hemsley, 1977).
Nevertheless, it should be noted that single-case methodology
is becoming a powerful tool for evaluating clinically based
treatment interventions.

The whole question of training parents to act as co-therapists
raises many problems which have been reviewed elsewhere (Yule,
1975; O'Dell, 1974). It is obviously important to learn which
parents with which sort of children can best benefit from the
sorts of approaches described here. If it is indeed true, as
Patterson (1975) believes, that one-third of the parents of
aggressive children can be helped by very simple interventions,
then it is a matter of urgency that such help should be readily
available in clinics in this country.

However, it is not a simple matter to transfer treatments that
have been found to be successful in one country and culture to
a different setting. Even treatment techniques can be situation
specific. British parents, by and large, do not expect to be
asked to read a programme text when they take their child to a
clinic. When they do read some of the American texts, they find
the language and the examples couched in alien jargon and slang.
But even when these factors are overcome, there is another cul-
tural difference which is often overlooked. This involves the
question of contingencies applied to parents.

Many of the American studies have been carried out from <u>research</u>
bases, rather than from <u>service</u> bases. In a country where treatment is not the right of all parents, and where treatment can be
prohibitively expensive, many parents may well agree to collec-
ting data in return for free advice on child management. Even
this sort of contingency contract (often implicit) has to be
strengthened. In some studies, parents have to put down a dep-
osit which is repaid in small sums as they complete assignments
or hand in data (Mira, 1970). In other studies, other material
reinforcers are dispersed (Johnson and Katz, 1973). Such management of clients appears foreign to British therapists, particularly because access to good treatment is the right of all
parents under our National Health Service.

Even so, given that conduct disorders have proved resistant to
other treatment approaches, it may well turn out that parents
have to be motivated by similar means to act as co-therapists.
Whatever the future holds, it is clear that the pioneering
American research in this area stands as an enormous challenge
to all of us offering help to children. Despite the problems
of transferring techniques from one culture to another, the
beauty of the behavioural approach lies in its problem-solving
philosophy. Transferring from Eugene to Ealing, or from Kansas
to Camberwell can be viewed as a problem of generalization
across stimulus settings and therefore it is potentially soluble!

It is inherent in a problem-solving approach that when limitations are observed, they will be viewed as obstacles to be overcome, rather than as necessary limits to be docilely accepted.
Behaviour modification has brought a new optimism to the treatment of conduct disorders. Future research will decide the extent to which such optimism may have to be qualified.

ACKNOWLEDGEMENTS

I would like to acknowledge my debt to Dr. Gerald Patterson,
Dr. Montrose Wolf, and their colleagues in Eugene, Oregon and
Lawrence, Kansas respectively, for the many hours of discussions
we shared. Acknowledgement is also due to the World Health
Organization who generously financed a Travelling Fellowship to
visit these projects in America.

REFERENCES

Alexander, J.F. and Parsons, B.V. (1973) Short-term behavioural
    intervention with delinquent families: Impact on family
    process and recidivism, J. Abnorm. Psychol. 81, 219-225.

Bandura, A. (1969) Principles of Behavior Modification. New
    York, Holt, Rinehart & Winston.

Bandura, A. (1973) Aggression: A Social Learning Analysis.
    London, Prentice Hall.

Bandura, A. and Walters, R.H. (1963) Social Learning and Per-
    sonality Development. New York, Holt, Rinehart & Winston.

Berkowitz, L. (1973) Control of aggression, in Caldwell, B.M.
    & Riciutti, H.N. (eds.), Review of Child Development Research
    Vol. 3. Child Development and Social Policy. University of
    Chicago Press.

Braukmann, C.J. and Fixsen, D.L. (1976) Behavior modification
    with delinquents, in Hersen, M., Eisler, R.M. & Miller, P.M.
    (eds.), Progress in Behavior Modification. New York, Academic
    Press.

Braukmann, C.J., Fixsen, D.L., Phillips, E.L., Wolf, M.M. and
    Maloney, D.M. (1974) An analysis of a selection interview
    training package for pre-delinquents at Achievement Place,
    Criminal Justice and Behavior, 1, 30-42.

Brown, P. and Elliott, R. (1965) Control of aggression in a nursery school class, J. Exper. Child Psychol. 2, 103-107.

Cautela, J.R. (1969) Behavior therapy and self-control: Techniques and implications, in Franks, C.M. (ed.), Behavior Therapy: Appraisal and Status. New York, McGraw Hill.

Cheyne, J.A. (1972) Punishment and "reasoning" in the development of self-control, in Parke, R.D. (ed.), Recent Trends in Social Learning Theory. New York, Academic Press.

Clark, H.B., Rowbury, T., Baer, A.M. and Baer, D.M. (1973) Time out as a punishing stimulus in continuous and intermittent schedules, J. Appl. Behav. Anal. 6, 443-455.

Clarke, R.V.G. and Cornish, D.B. (1976) The effectiveness of residential treatment for delinquents. (This volume).

Clarke, R.V.G. and Martin, D.N. (1971) Absconding from Approved Schools. London, H.M.S.O.

Cohen H.L. and Filipczak, J. (1971) A New Learning Environment. San Francisco, Jossey-Bass.

Cornish, D.B. and Clarke, R.V.G. (1975) Residential Treatment and its Effects on Delinquency. London, H.M.S.O.

Davidson, W.S. and Seidman, E. (1974) Studies of behavior modification and juvenile delinquency: A review, methodological critique and social perspective, Psychol. Bull. 81, 998-1011.

Dawe, H.C. (1934) An analysis of two hundred quarrels of pre-school children, Child Devel. 5, 139-157.

Eitzen, D.S. (1975) The effects of behavior modification on the attitudes of delinquents, Behav. Res. Ther. 13, 295-299.

Eyberg, S.M. and Johnson, S.M. (1974) Multiple assessment of behavior modification with families, J. Consult. Clin. Psychol. 42, 594-606.

Ferber, H. Keeley, S.M. and Shemberg, K.M (1974) Training parents in behavior modification: Outcome of and problems encountered in a program after Patterson's work, Behav. Ther. 5, 415-419.

Forehand, R., King, H.E., Peed, S. and Yoder, P. (1975). Mother-child interactions: comparison of a non-compliant clinic group and a non-clinic group, Behav. Res. Ther. 13, 79-84.

Hops, H. and Walters, R.H. (1963) Studies of reinforcement of aggression: II - Effects of emotionally-arousing antecedent conditions, Child Devel. 34, 553-562.

Johnson, C.A. and Katz, R.C. (1973) Using parents as change agents for their children: A review, J. Child Psychol. Psychiatr. 14, 181-200.

Johnson, S.M. and Lobitz, G.K. (1974) Parental manipulation of child behavior in home observations, J. Appl. Behav. Anal. 7, 23-31.

Kifer, R.E., Lewis, M.A., Green, D.R. and Phillips, E.L. (1974) Training predelinquent youths and their parents to negotiate conflict situations, J. Appl. Behav. Anal. 7, 357-364.

MacDonough, T.S. and Forehand, R. (1973) Response-contingent time out: Important factors in behavior modification with children, J. Behav. Ther. Exper. Psychiat. 4, 231-236.

Matthews, A. (1975) Research design and clinical practice in behaviour therapy, Brit. Ass. Behav. Psychother. Bull. 3, 43-46.

Mira, M. (1970) Results of a behavior modification training program for parents and teachers, Behav. Res. Ther. 8, 309-311.

O'Dell, S. (1974) Training parents in behaviour modification: A review, Psychol. Bull. 81, 418-433.

O'Leary, K.D. and O'Leary, S.G. (eds.), (1972) Classroom Management: The Successful Use of Behavior Modification. Oxford, Pergamon.

Patterson, G.R. (1965) Responsiveness to social stimuli, in Krasner, L. & Ullmann, L.P. (eds.), Research in Behavior Modification. New York, Holt, Rinehart & Winston.

Patterson, G.R. (1969) Behavioral techniques based upon social learning: An additional base for developing behavior modification technologies, in Franks, C.M. (ed.), Behavior Therapy: Appraisal and Status. New York, McGraw Hill.

Patterson, G.R. (1971) Families: Applications of Social Learning Theory to Family Life. Champaign, Ill., Research Press.

Patterson, G.R. (1974a) Interventions for boys with conduct problems: Multiple settings, treatments and criteria, J. Consult. Clin. Psychol. 42, 471-481.

Patterson, G.R. (1974b) Multiple evaluations of a parent training program, in Thompson, T. (ed.), Proceedings of the First International Symposium on Behavior Modification. New York, Appleton-Century-Crofts.

Patterson, G.R. (1974c) Retraining of aggressive boys by their parents: Review of recent literature and follow-up evaluation, Canad. Psychiat. Assoc. J., 19, 142-161.

Patterson, G.R. (1975) The aggressive child: Victim and architect of a coercive system, in Hamerlynck, L.A., Mash, E.J. & Handy, L.C. (eds.), Behavior Modification and Families. New York, Brunner Mazel.

Patterson, G.R. and Brodsky, G. (1966) A behaviour modification programme for a child with multiple problem behaviour, J. Child Psychol. Psychiat. 7, 277-295.

Patterson, G.R. and Cobb, J.A. (1971) A dyadic analysis of aggressive behavior, in Hill, J.P. (ed.), Minnesota Symposia on Child Psychology, Vol. 5. Minneapolis, Univ. Minnesota Press.

Patterson, G.R., Cobb, J.A. and Ray, R.S. (1972) Direct intervention in the classroom: A set of procedures for the aggressive child, in Clark, F., Evans, D. & Hamerlynck, L. (eds.), Implementing Behavioral Programs for Schools and Clinics. Champaign, Ill., Research Press.

Patterson, G.R., Cobb, J.A. and Ray, R.S. (1973) A social engineering technology for retraining the families of aggressive boys, in Adams, H.E. & Unikel, I.P. (eds.), Issues and Trends in Behavior Therapy. Springfield, Ill., Charles C. Thomas.

Patterson, G.R. and Gullion, M.E. (1968) Living with Children: New Methods for Parents and Teachers. Champaign, Ill., Research Press.

Patterson, G.R., Littman, R.A. and Bricker, W. (1967) Assertive
behavior in children: A step towards a theory of aggression,
Monogr. Soc. Res. Child. Dev. 32(5), Series No. 113.

Patterson, G.R. and Reid, J.B. (1970) Reciprocity and coercion:
Two facets of social systems, in Neuringer, C. & Michael, J.
(eds.), Behavior Modification in Clinical Psychology. New
York, Appleton Century Crofts.

Patterson, G.R. and Reid, J.B. (1973) Intervention for families
of aggressive boys: A replication study, Behav. Res. Ther.
11, 383-394.

Patterson, G.R., Weiss, R.L. and Hops, H. (1975) Training of
marital skills: Some problems and concepts, in Leitenberg, H.
(ed.), Handbook of Operant Techniques. New York, Prentice-
Hall.

Phillips, E.A., Phillips, E.L., Fixsen, D.L. and Wolf, M.M. (1976)
Achievement Place: The training of social skills, J. Appl.
Behav. Anal. (in press).

Phillips, E.L. (1968) Achievement Place: token reinforcement
procedures in a home-style rehabilitation setting for predelinquent boys, J. Appl. Behav. Anal. 1, 213-223.

Phillips, E.L., Phillips, E.A., Fixsen, D.L. and Wolf. M.M. (1972)
The Teaching-Family Handbook. Lawrence, Kansas, University
of Kansas.

Phillips, E.L., Phillips, E.A., Fixsen, D.L. and Wolf, M.M. (1973)
Behavior shaping works with delinquents, Psychology Today,
June.

Reid, J. and Hendricks, A.F.C.J. (1973) Preliminary analysis
of the effectiveness of direct home intervention for the
treatment of predelinquent boys who steal, in Hamerlynck,
L.A., Handy, L.C. & Mash, E.J. (eds.), Behavior Change:
Methodology, Concepts and Practice. Champaign, Ill., Research
Press.

Robins, L.N. (1966) Deviant Children Grown Up. Baltimore,
Williams & Wilkins.

Ross A.O. (1974) Psychological Disorders of Children: A
Behavioral Approach to Theory, Research and Therapy. New
York, McGraw-Hill.

Rutter, M. and Yule, W. (1970) Reading retardation and anti-
social behavior - the nature of the association. in Rutter, M.,
Tizard, J. & Whitmore, K. (eds.), Education, Health and
Behaviour. London, Longmans.

Sachs, D.A. (1973) The efficacy of time-out procedures in a
variety of behavior problems, J. Behav. Ther. and Exper.
Psychiat. 4, 237-242.

Sherman, J.A. and Bushell, D. (1975) Behaviour modification as
an educational technique, in Horowitz, F.D. (ed.), Review of
Child Development Research, Vol. 4. University of Chicago
Press.

Staats, A.W. and Butterfield, W.H. (1965) Treatment of non-
reading in a culturally-deprived juvenile delinquent: An
application of reinforcement principles, Child Devel. 36,
925-942.

Tharp, R. and Wetzel, R. (1969) Behavior Modification in the
Natural Environment. New York, Academic Press.

Thoresen, C. (ed.), (1973) Behavior Modification in Education.
72nd Year Book, National Society for the Study of Education,
U.S.A.

Thoresen, C.E. and Mahoney, M.J. (1974) Behavioral Self-Control.
New York, Holt-Rinehart.

Walter, H. and Gilmore, S.K. (1973) Placebo versus social learning effects in parent training procedures designed to alter
the behavior of aggressive boys, Behav. Ther. 4, 361-377.

Walters, R.H., Cheyne, J.A. and Banks, R.K. (1972) Punishment.
Harmondsworth, Penguin.

Ward, J. (1975) Behaviour modification in special education,
in Wedell, K. (ed.), Orientations in Special Education.
London, Wiley.

Wiltz, N.A. and Patterson, G.R. (1974) An evaluation of parent
training procedures designed to alter inappropriate aggressive behaviors of boys, Behav. Ther. 5, 515-521.

Wolf, M.M., Phillips, E.L. and Fixsen, D.L. (1975) Achievement
Place Phase II: Final Report. Dept. of Human Development,
Univ. Kansas.

Yule, W. (1975) Teaching psychological principles to non-psychologists: Training parents in child management, J. Ass. Educ. Psychol. 10, 5-16.

Yule, W. (1976) Behavioural treatment of children's disorders, Psikijatrija Danas (Psychiatry Today, Belgrade), 8, 173-190.

Yule, W. (1977a) Behavioural approaches to treatment, in Rutter, M. & Hersov, L. (eds.), Child Psychiatry: Modern Approaches. London, Blackwell Scientific Publications.

Yule, W. (1977b) Observation and recording techniques, Chapter 2, in Yule, W. & Carr, J. (eds.), A Course on Behaviour Modification with the Severely Retarded (to be published).

Yule, W. (1977c) Evaluation of treatment programmes, Chapter 10 in Yule, W. & Carr, J. (eds.), A Course on Behaviour Modification with the Severely Retarded (to be published).

Yule, W. and Hemsley, D. (1977) Single case methodology in medical psychology, in Rachman, S. (ed.), Advances in Medical Psychology. Oxford, Pergamon.

THE EFFECTIVENESS OF RESIDENTIAL
TREATMENT FOR DELINQUENTS

R. V. G. Clarke and D. B. Cornish

INTRODUCTION

Delinquent children who repeatedly come to the attention of the authorities tend in this country to end up in some form of residential care. This will normally be provided in a community home with education on the premises which, prior to the implementation of the Children and Young Persons Act 1969, would have been known as an approved school. In March 1975 approximately 6400 children were in residence at these institutions. This paper attempts to present a balanced view of the effectiveness of such residential treatment in bringing about a long-term reduction in delinquency. It begins by briefly discussing a controlled trial recently completed by the authors of the differential effectiveness of two residential programmes. The negative results reported from this research are shown to be consistent with the findings from most other studies in this field. It is concluded that different institutional programmes give similar results and that overall success at "curing" delinquency is low. An explanation for this failure is attempted and alternative modes of treatment are discussed. Lastly, some suggestions for improving existing institutional practice are given. Though the paper is pessimistic about the role of residential treatment in reducing recividism it is recognized that these institutions may serve other roles such as care, control and general deterrence: these are briefly described at the end of the paper.

"Treatment" in community homes with education on the premises usually means the provision of a structured regime where, during a carefully ordered day, boys are provided with education, organized leisure and, if they are old enough, some basic training in trades such as gardening, carpentry or decorating. Pastoral care is usually organized on a house basis, where house-parents (who normally live in) are responsible for boys' welfare and for the liaison with their homes and field social workers. Before placement in the community home, boys are of course likely to have received comprehensive social, educational, psychological and psychiatric assessments (Ostapuik and Porteous, 1974) at residential assessment centres, but subsequent treat-

143

ment is rarely able to match the sophistication of their recom-
mendations. In addition to their diagnostic role, psychiatrists
are also employed on a sessional basis by many of the community
homes to which the boys are sent. Limitations on the time available, together with the apparent unsuitability of most of the
boys for individual psychotherapy, have led both psychiatrists
(Evans, 1963) and the homes' staff (Heads' Association, 1968) to
place greater emphasis upon other areas of psychiatric involvement, such as providing training, advice and support for staff
in their dealings with the boys.

During the 1950s, however, developments in group therapeutic
techniques made it possible to extend the treatment side in
approved schools, and various attempts to adapt the most thor-
ough-going of these approaches — the therapeutic community (Jones,
1952)— to the residential treatment of delinquents were made
(Craft et al., 1964; Wills, 1971; McMichael, 1972; Cornish
and Clarke, 1975). In the United States experimentation took a
similar course, though the variety of therapeutic techniques was
somewhat greater; there, institutions have been run on the lines
of guided group interaction (Weeks, 1958; Empey and Rabow, 1961),
"reality" therapy, transactional analysis (Jesness et al., 1972),
token economies (Kazdin and Bootzin, 1972), and other behaviour
modification systems such as contingency contracting (Jesness
et al., 1972) as well as by breaking large institutions down
into smaller units (Jesness, 1965) or integrating them more
fully into the neighbouring community (Empey and Lubeck, 1971).

Evaluative research in relation to the institutional treatment
of juveniles has generally taken the form of a comparison between
one or more of these innovations and an existing approach. Equi-
valence of intake between the treatments being compared is en-
sured by the use of random allocation, matching, or prediction
techniques, and success is evaluated in terms of further offending after release.

AN EXAMPLE OF EVALUATIVE RESEARCH: THE KINGSWOOD CONTROLLED TRIAL

A recent study conducted by the authors (cf. Cornish and Clarke,
1975) of a "therapeutic community" established in one of the
three houses of Kingswood Training School, a West Country
approved school catering for boys aged 13-15 on admission, is
illustrative of existing evaluative research. The therapeutic
community, which had been developed by a resident psychologist,

was based on four principles (cf. Rapoport, 1960): the sharing
of responsibility between staff and boys for making decisions
on matters of common concern (democratization); the creation
of an informal atmosphere such that, for example, staff shared
some domestic duties with the boys and were known by their
christian names (communalism); the toleration of a wide measure
of "acting out" behaviour (permissiveness); and the continuous
attempt to communicate to boys the ways in which others interpreted their behaviour (reality confrontation). The main vehicles
of treatment were the twice-daily meetings of the whole community, when day-to-day problems of group living were discussed,
and smaller groups of boys and staff which met once or twice a
week to discuss individual problems. Attempts were also made to
utilize the therapeutic potential of other aspects of house life,
such as domestic duties. Because of the controversy surrounding
what was then a new form of treatment for approved schools, the
school's Managers decided that an evaluation of the regime should
be attempted.

Research Method

The research design was intended to allow the staff of the therapeutic community some measure of choice in the boys they attempted to treat, while ensuring at the same time that a valid comparison could be made with the treatment offered in the rest of
the school. It was decided that those judged suitable for the
therapeutic community (an estimated two-thirds of the boys admitted to the school) would be randomly assigned on admission between the therapeutic community and a "control" house which had
a well-established regime run on traditional, paternalistic
lines. Boys judged unsuitable were allocated to the school's
third house. The main finding from subsequent analysis of a
wide range of background factors was that these boys were of
significantly lower IQ (mean 91.4 compared with a mean of 104.5
for the "suitable" boys).

The controlled trial was in operation for about 4 years, during
which time 280 boys were assigned between the three houses of
the school. A detailed study of the regimes showed therapeutic
community staff to be more treatment-oriented — in overall
ideology, in attitudes and in policies — than those in the control house. Differences in behaviour between the groups of boys
in the two houses being compared were also in the expected direction: boys in the therapeutic community, for instance, were
more likely to act out by absconding or by damaging the furni-
ture and fabric of the house.

Each boy was followed-up for 2 years after release through the Criminal Records Office in order to obtain information about further offending.

Results

No differences were found between the therapeutic community and the control house in the number of boys convicted during the two years immediately following their stay in the school (Table 1). Table 1 also shows that there were no differences between these two houses and the third house receiving the "unsuitable" boys.

TABLE 1

Reconvictions of Boys Taking Part in the Kingswood Study

House	Number admitted	Number reconvicted	% reconvicted
Therapeutic community	86	60	70%
"Control" house	87	60	69%
Third house	107	73	68%
All boys	280	193	69%

Results such as these tend to be questioned — especially if attempts are made to generalize from the findings — on the grounds that implementation of the experimental treatment may have been inadequate. The extent to which this criticism was justified in the present research has been fully discussed elsewhere (Cornish and Clarke, 1975), as has the issue of generalizing from results (Clarke and Cornish, 1972). In order to cast some light on both these points, the reconviction rates of two other schools served by the same regional assessment centre as Kingswood Training School and which, during the latter part of the research, also began to operate as therapeutic communities were studied. These were found not to differ from the reconviction rates of the three houses at Kingswood.

PREVIOUS RESEARCH FINDINGS

(a)   The Criterion of Reconviction

As will be shown later, negative findings, like those of the
Kingswood research, are characteristic of much of the evaluative
research in this field, and it will be argued that this has
implications for theories and methods of treating delinquents.
This being so, it is necessary at the outset to deal with one
criticism frequently raised by proponents of residential treatment: that reconviction is not an adequate measure of success
and may not even be a relevant one.

Staff are accustomed to seeing boys settle down in their institution, put on weight, improve their reading, and become able
to be taken off tranquillizing drugs during their stay. They
inevitably feel that these successes are not adequately reflected
in the crude statistics of reconviction rates. Not only, so
the argument goes, are the offences which make up these statistics often trivial but, more importantly, evidence of subsequent
delinquency in the relatively short-term is not necessarily a
relevant criterion. Advocates of this view stress that it is
more important to know whether a boy is emotionally adjusted or
whether he can make successful relationships and hold down a
job, and that it is necessary to extend the period of follow-up
into adulthood to obtain a more balanced picture.

Unfortunately, however, improvements in a boy's health, education
and general wellbeing during his stay are no guarantee that his
delinquent conduct will be reduced as a result. Moreover, quite
apart from the fact that offenders are sent to institutions as
a consequence of their delinquency (and, therefore, presumably
to be "cured"), it is difficult to see how long-term personal
adjustment — however defined — can be achieved without an improvement in delinquency. Indeed, several investigations (Glueck and
Glueck, 1934; Scott, 1964; Hood, 1966) indicate that post-
treatment recidivism is associated with continuing poor adjustment in many other areas of a person's life. Finally, longer
periods of follow-up provide even more depressing figures concerning recidivism — Hammond (1968) found that of the 254 senior
approved school boys whom he followed up for nine years, 60%
became continuous and persistent offenders and about 40% had
received sentences of imprisonment as adults.

(b)   The Effectiveness of Residential Intervention in Reducing Delinquency

As mentioned above, the Kingswood results are consistent with the generality of research in this field. As far as British studies are concerned, McMichael (1974) found no significant differences in the reconviction rates of boys from a Scottish approved school run as a therapeutic community and a control group of boys from other schools. Craft et al.'s (1964) study of authoritarian and permissive regimes for adolescent psychopaths found no differences between them in numbers of boys subsequently offending and Craft's (1965) study of an exceptionally well organized "family-type" programme in one approved school for junior boys showed that it achieved no better than average success. With older offenders, Bottoms and McClintock (1973) found that two different borstal regimes — one giving traditional, the other more individualized training — produced similar reconviction rates.

A pattern of predominantly negative findings also exists in American research: differential outcomes have not emerged from the important studies of the last few years which have dealt with juvenile delinquents and which have utilized some method of satisfactorily matching inputs to the programmes being compared (e.g. Jesness, 1971; Empey and Lubeck, 1971; Jesness et al., 1972). In those cases (e.g. the original Highfields research of Weeks, 1958, and Jesness's Fricot Ranch Study, 1965) where differences in outcome were found, there is considerable doubt about the validity of the results because of breakdowns in, or lack of, adequate input matching. It may be worth noting in passing that reviews of American evaluative research into institutional treatment for adult offenders have also failed to show evidence of differential effectiveness (Morris, 1971; Robison and Smith, 1971; Martinson, 1974; and Brody, 1976). Moreover, the lack of firm evidence concerning any differential effects of different institutional programmes needs to be seen in the context of the low overall levels of success achieved: the 70% reconviction rate observed at Kingswood (which, because only a small proportion of offences is detected, almost certainly underestimates the true level of offending) is fairly typical for approved schools (H.M.S.O., 1972).

Small differences in effectiveness between different institutional regimes have been found, however, in two recent studies (Dunlop, 1975; Sinclair and Clarke, 1973) which used "cross-institutional" designs. Instead of making comparisons between

only two or three different institutional treatments as in the
normal designs, such studies take a larger number of institutions
and correlate measures of effectiveness with measures of particular aspects of the treatment process. It has been argued
(Clarke and Sinclair, 1973) that insofar as a large number of
comparisons are made simultaneously, these designs are especially
useful in finding which specific components of the treatment
situation are likely to be the effective ones.

In her study, Dunlop (1975) measured the emphasis placed by
eight approved schools catering for boys aged between 13 and 15
on the following regime components: education; trade training;
leisure; staff, other adult, and peer relationships; maturity
and responsibility; religion; punishment and deterrence.
Having re-ordered the reconviction rates of the schools to take
account of differing intakes, she then correlated the regime
emphasis scores with five-year reconviction rates for the schools
concerned. One of the principal findings of the research was
that schools which emphasized trade training had lower reconviction rates. This may not, however, have been because of the
trade training provided, but because of the better behaviour
and lower rates of absconding in these schools: Sinclair and
Clarke (1973) had found earlier in their cross-institutional
study of 66 approved schools that reconviction rates were significantly correlated with absconding rates, even when differences
among intakes to the school had been allowed for. They argued
that these results showed that "acting out" problems by absconding was not generally therapeutic but merely provided boys with
fresh opportunities to commit delinquent acts and, as a consequence, to further establish delinquent patterns of response.

Such marginal effects could only be detected through cross-
institutional designs, and for this reason more weight should
be given to the negative results of the evaluative research
reported earlier. Moreover, while providing evidence against
the suggestion that nothing that institutional programmes do,
or omit to do, makes any difference to the subsequent delinquency
of their charges, cross-institutional studies still fail to provide evidence that some programmes are more effective at reducing
post-treatment delinquency than others. It may rather be that
programmes described as "better" are merely those whose effects
are neutral rather than beneficial.

(c) The Impact of Institutional Environment on Current
Behaviour

Cross-institutional designs are more important, not for showing
the small differences in post-release reconviction rates which
may occur, but for indicating the very large differences which
exist between institutions in the behaviour they elicit from
similar types of residents while these are still in their care.
In the first of these studies (Sinclair, 1971), though (with
one exception) no differences were found between the reconviction rates of the probation hostels studied, there were very
marked differences (ranging from 14% to 78%) in their "drop-out"
rates as a result of absconding or further offending. (A recent
study by Tutt (1976) indicates that "drop-out" rates for
community homes with education on the premises show similar
variations (from 15% to 66%).) Sinclair was able to show that
the variation in drop-out rates was not due to differences in
the boys admitted to the various probation hostels, nor could
it be accounted for by the more obvious features of the hostel:
the differences between successive wardens in the same hostel
were as wide as those between wardens in different hostels and
there was no association with the size, age range or location
of hostels. A detailed study of hostel regimes showed, however,
that those with low drop-out rates were characterized by a
strict regime where the warden had related closely to the boys
in his charge and was in agreement with his wife about the way
the hostel should be run. Those who were harsh, emotionally
distant, lax or who disagreed with their wives about hostel pol-
icy tended to have high drop-out rates from their hostels.

Cross-institutional studies as detailed as Sinclair's (1971)
study have not been carried out in approved schools or community
homes, but Clarke and Martin (1971) have shown that the very
marked differences in absconding which exist between approved
schools (ranging, for example, from 10% to 75% of the populations
in individual senior approved schools) cannot be accounted for
by differences in boys admitted and must be the result of exposure to differing school environments. From limited studies
undertaken in one or two schools they were able to show that
amount of absconding was related to the recency and circumstances
of a boy's admission and the recency of his return from leave.
It was also more common when it had not recently been dealt with
by corporal punishment. Though resources did not permit a more
detailed study of the regime factors implicated in absconding,
the authors argued in the report that any event that produced
even temporary unhappiness or insecurity in a boy could lead to

absconding and that the more opportunities to abscond provided
by the regime, the more absconding there would be. There was
also evidence that certain boys developed a habit of absconding
and that some schools could either facilitate or inhibit the
development of this.

EXPLAINING THE INEFFECTIVENESS OF RESIDENTIAL TREATMENT

It might reasonably be asked how it is that, since institutional
environments appear to have such a marked influence upon the
current behaviour of their charges, this effect does not persist
after the boys leave. Far from being inconsistent with one another, the two sets of research findings reviewed in the previous
section can be interpreted as indicating that whilst any environment is an important determinant of its inhabitants' current
behaviour, this influence will persist only so long as they
remain within that, or a similar, setting. When boys move from
community homes into the post-institutional environment,
therefore, their behaviour will become subject to a different
set of situational stimuli which, unlike those of the institution, may elicit delinquent behaviour.

But existing residential treatments see delinquency as being
largely the expression of longstanding anti-social attitudes and
maladjusted personality (genetic in origin or the product of
early learning experiences). This is not to say that the individual's current environment is accorded no attention. Attempts
are made, for example, to improve family relationships and provide the boy with a job on leaving. But residential staff have
relatively few opportunities to intervene in the home environment and relatively little faith that by so doing they will be
tackling the major source of behavioural variance — this is seen
as residing within the individual. In other words, a "medical
model" of delinquency and its treatment underlies much current
residential practice.

This medical model of delinquency and its treatment has come
increasingly under fire in recent years from two directions.
Firstly, sociologists of the "deviancy" school have argued that
those who view delinquency simply as a disorder of individual
functioning, have tended to ignore three things: the fact that
it is society which defines particular behaviours as delinquent;
that different societies (and different social groups within a
society) may accord varying degrees of opprobrium to particular

forms of behaviour; and that, this being the case, it is likely
that those forms of behaviour disapproved of by the more powerful or influential segments of society, will be the ones labelled
as delinquent and proscribed by the criminal law. Commentators
(Chapman, 1968) have also called attention — perhaps as a corol-
lary to the last point — to the bias, witting or unwitting, in
the enforcement of laws which disproportionately singles out the
poor or disadvantaged for punishment and thus for definition as
criminal or delinquent. This despite the evidence of self-report
studies of delinquent conduct which have shown that, since even
serious delinquency is quite widespread in the population, it
is incorrect to treat it as being the prerogative of a highly
abnormal minority of disordered individuals. In the light of
these findings, it is perhaps not surprising that several decades
of careful psychological research have seen little success in
establishing clear-cut personality differences between those who
commit crimes and those who do not. Some differences have indeed been found, but these are not marked and can often be explained by the effects of incarceration.

The failure to identify personality traits characteristic of
criminals is consistent with a general lack of success, in the
wider field of psychology, to show clear relationships between
measures of personality on the one hand and behaviour on the
other. Mischel (1968) has argued in much greater detail than
is possible here that if highly generalized personality traits
were important in determining behaviour then there should be
much greater consistency of behaviour over time and across a
variety of situations than the available research suggests.
Far from demonstrating that an individual tends to respond in a
characteristic manner in different situations and at different
times, however, research suggests on the contrary that a person's
behaviour is heavily influenced by the immediate situation in
which he finds himself. As far as delinquency is concerned,
Hartshorne and May (1928) showed in a classic study nearly 50
years ago that children who (given the opportunity) behave del-
inquently in a particular situation may not do so when placed
in even a slightly different one. Their research was carried
out under experimental conditions, but its implication is that
any attempt to explain and, arguably, to treat delinquency
without paying due regard to the strong influence of the individual's immediate social and physical environment will not
meet with success.

It also calls attention to the highly specific nature of the
circumstances and conditions that can give rise to delinquent

behaviour. Thus for a particular boy the significant factors
may be that his parents allow him too much freedom to wander the
streets (Wilson, 1975); or that his school has thrown him into
contact with a group of boys who gain status from shoplifting;
or that the neglected city environment he inhabits may provide
limitless opportunities for vandalism and burglary; or that
support of the local football club may provide the ready occa-
sion for hooliganism; or the fact that he cannot read or write
may lead him to use his motorcycle without tax or insurance.
Such a list could be greatly lengthened and, of course, particular boys may be exposed to a wide range of unfavourable environmental circumstances.

That delinquent conduct persists might be explained by the fact
that the individual's environment has not altered or that he has
developed specifically delinquent modes of response to the environmental stimuli. There is therefore a ready explanation for
the failure of any treatment which pays insufficient regard to
these environmental pressures or that does not attempt to deal
directly with them. No amount of exposure within a residential
setting to "casework", to "therapeutic" relationships or, more
simply, to a disciplined and structured regime is likely to have
much effect if the boy is thereafter returned to his home environment with its familiar pressures and inducements to delinquent
conduct.

ALTERNATIVE TREATMENTS

There is insufficient space in this paper to discuss the treatment implications of a view which emphasizes the role of specific environmental contingencies in delinquency causation and,
indeed, these have yet to be fully worked out. It would seem,
however, that treatment or — to use what is perhaps a more
appropriate term — intervention, will usually have to take place
in the delinquent's normal environment. This should not, however, be taken as endorsement of current non-custodial treatments, many of which in practice also operate on an "inner
causality" model of delinquency and which have not been shown
to be any more successful than institutional programmes (Harlow,
1970; Martinson, 1974). It could consist, rather, of (1)
attempts to modify the specific features of the child's environment that provide the impetus for his delinquency; (2) the
imposition of selective controls on his movements to restrict
the opportunities for delinquency; (3) the application of
behaviour modification techniques (making use, perhaps, of his

parents or teachers) to change specific delinquent habits; and
(4) training in social or educational skills where their defi-
ciency is related to the child's delinquency or where they might
produce realistic alternative ways of responding. Far from con-
stituting a naively behaviouristic and anti-individualistic
approach, such methods emphasize once again two essential pre-
requisites of individual treatment: (1) the careful and detailed
analysis of the behaviour patterns of individuals — a consideration which should particularly appeal to the clinician (Cliffe
et al., 1974); and (2) the primacy of the individual case, in
the sense that treatment must be accurately fitted to his requirements and not the organizational aims of existing institutions
and their staff — to continue, to keep full, to remain unchanged.

How far such a model is practicable has yet to be determined,
though certain treatment developments in the United States are
consistent with the approach (cf. Yule, p. 115 of this volume).
As delinquents would remain in the community for treatment,
the public may in practice have to be somewhat more tolerant of
the persistent offending of certain children while at the same
time accepting the degree of intervention in children's lives
that treatment would sometimes involve (though this would be
less than is involved in removing them to a community home).
Social workers would have to be trained in behaviour modification and other specialist skills and they would need to espouse
a more active interventionist role than the traditional one of
making relationships, providing advice and support, and occasional practical assistance. Fresh legislation might be needed
in order to furnish the necessary powers to impose selective
restrictions on a child's freedom of movement and the system as
a whole would require substantial resources that in practice
might be judged appropriate for only a small proportion of cases
— though it should not be forgotten that the present system of
institutional treatment is also very expensive.

THE IMMEDIATE FUTURE OF RESIDENTIAL TREATMENT

This paper has confined its attention principally to the issue
of whether institutional treatment is an effective instrument
for reducing delinquent behaviour in the long-term. As a result
of their own and a large body of other evaluative research, the
authors have concluded not only that residential placement does
not serve this purpose, but that it cannot.

There are those, however, who will argue that the institutions

have other functions, and that proposals to re-allocate resources
to other forms of intervention must first take proper account of
these. Little empirical investigation has been done, for example,
of the belief that sending persistent offenders to community
homes acts as a deterrent to other children, though the existence
of such an effect might have important implications for the
question of how far resource re-allocation should go. Again, it
is likely that persistently delinquent children will continue to
be sent to community homes, if only because there may appear to
be no other way of providing them with the care and control they
need. Whether either of these needs has to be, or indeed is,
served by placement in a residential institution might itself be
made the subject of detailed and regular study: levels of absconding in community homes (cf. Tutt, 1976) and in approved
schools before them (Clarke and Martin, 1971) suggest, as a start,
that neither requirement is as well served as it might be.

Despite the analysis offered above it is likely that many of the
institutions will retain treatment ambitions and while at best
only very marginal increments in success are likely to be
achieved, existing research does contain pointers to more effective practice. First, trade training seems to be valued by boys
(Dunlop, 1975; Millham et al., 1975) and schools which appear
to emphasize this have been found to be slightly more successful
than others (Dunlop, 1975), though whether their success was due
to trade training itself is arguable, since they also laid stress
on responsible conduct within the school and generally had lower
rates of absconding. Second, "therapeutic communities" or regimes in which attempts are made to foster closer "casework" relationships between staff and children have not shown any marked
degree of success, while there is evidence from research in
probation hostels (Sinclair, 1971) that it is particularly difficult to combine closer relationships with the degree of firmness
that is necessary in dealing with delinquents. In sum, therefore,
the existing research indicates that institutions which are run
in a firm (but not harsh) way, where there is little absconding
and where (perhaps) trade training is emphasized, may be margin-
ally more effective in the long term than others. While attempts
to do so have not been very successful to date, it might also be
that those institutions which pay close attention to a boy's transition back to his own home and to the situation he will encounter
there would achieve somewhat greater success — though this shift
in emphasis would itself implicitly recognize both the limited
usefulness of residential aspects of treatment, and the importance of the boy's natural environment. Because of this, such
improvements must be seen as making the best of the present

unsatisfactory and in many ways irrelevent system. Tinkering with institutional machinery should not be allowed to deflect the search for ways of treating delinquents within the community, making use of knowledge concerning the powerful determinants of delinquent conduct in the individual's immediate social and physical environment.

REFERENCES

Bottoms, A.E. and McClintock, F.H. (1973) Criminals Coming of Age. London, Heinemann.

Brody, S.R. (1976) The Effectiveness of Sentencing - A Review of the Literature. London, H.M.S.O.

Chapman, D. (1968) Sociology and the Stereotype of the Criminal. London, Tavistock Publications.

Clarke, R.V.G. and Cornish, D.B. (1972) The Controlled Trial in Institutional Research - Paradigm or Pitfall for Penal Evaluators? London, H.M.S.O.

Clarke, R.V.G. and Martin, D.N. (1971) Absconding from Approved Schools. London, H.M.S.O.

Clarke, R.V.G. and Sinclair, I.A.C. (1973) Towards more effective treatment evaluation, Paper to First Criminological Colloquium, Council of Europe: Strasbourg.

Cliffe, M.J., Gathercole, C. and Epling, W.F. (1974) Some implications of the experimental analysis of behaviour for behaviour modification, Bull. Brit. Psychol. Soc. 27, 390-397.

Cornish, D.B. and Clarke, R.V.G. (1975) Residential Treatment and its Effects on Delinquency. London, H.M.S.O.

Craft, M. (1965) A follow up study of disturbed juvenile delinquents, Brit. J. Crim. 5, 55-62.

Craft, M., Stephenson, G. and Granger, C. (1964) A controlled trial of authoritarian and self governing regimes with adolescent psychopaths, Amer. J. Orthopsychiat. 34, 543-554.

Dunlop, A. (1975) The Approved School Experience. London, H.M.S.O.

Empey, L.T. and Lubeck, S.G. (1971) The Silverlake Experiment: Testing Delinquency Theory and Community Intervention. Chicago, Aldine Publishing Co.

Empey, L.T. and Rabow, J. (1961) The Provo experiment in delinquency rehabilitation, Amer. Sociol. Rev. 26, 679-696.

Evans, J. (1963) Has the psychiatrist a useful function in an approved school? Brit. J. Criminol. 4, 127-144.

Glueck, S. and Glueck, E.T. (1934) One Thousand Delinquents: Their Treatment by Court and Clinic, (Reprinted 1965). New York, Kraus Reprint Corporation.

Hammond, W.H. (1968) Research into the subsequent histories of a sample of ex-approved school boys, Paper to a meeting of Approved School Psychologists, Sunningdale.

Harlow, E. (1970) Intensive intervention: an alternative to institutionalization, Crime and Delinquen. Lit. 2, 3-46.

Hartshorne, H. and May, M.A. (1928) Studies in Deceit, Vol. 1 of Studies in the Nature of Character. New York, Macmillan.

Heads' Association (1968) The need for psychiatric treatment within the approved schools, Memorandum prepared by the Technical Sub-Committee of the Association of Headmasters, Headmistresses and Matrons of Approved Schools, Approved Schools Gazette, 62, 16-22.

H.M.S.O. (1972) Statistics relating to Approved Schools, Remand Homes and Attendance Centres in England and Wales for the year 1970. London, H.M.S.O.

Hood, R.G. (1966) Homeless Borstal Boys: A Study of their After-Care and After Conduct. Occasional Papers on Social Administration, No. 18. London, Bell & Sons.

Jesness, C.F. (1965) The Fricot Ranch Study. California Department of the Youth Authority (mimeo).

Jesness, C.F. (1971) The Preston Typology Study: An experiment with differential treatment in an institution, J. Res. Crime Delinquen. 8, 38-52.

Jesness, C.F., DeRisi, W.J., McCormick, P.M. and Wedge, R.F. (1972) The Youth Centre Research Project. California, American Justice Institute in co-operation with California Youth Authority (mimeo).

Jones, M. (1952) Social Psychiatry. London, Tavistock Publications.

Kazdin, A.E. and Bootzin, R.R. (1972) The token economy: an evaluative review, J. Appl. Behav. Anal. 5, 343-372.

Martinson, R. (1974) What works? - questions and answers about prison reform, The Public Interest, Spring, 22-34.

McMichael, P. (1972) Loaningdale School - A Study of the Impact of an Experimental Regime. Social Work Services Group, Scotland (copies obtainable from the author).

McMichael, P. (1974) After-care, family relationships, and re-conviction in a Scottish approved school, Brit. J. Criminol. 14, 236-247.

Millham, S., Bullock, R. and Cherrett, P. (1975) After Grace - Teeth: A Comparative Study of the Residential Experience of Boys in Approved Schools. London, Chaucer Publishing Co. Ltd.

Mischel, W. (1968) Personality and Assessment. New York, Wiley.

Morris, A. (1971) A correctional administrator's guide to the evaluation of correctional programs, Correctional Research, No. 21, Boston Massachusetts Correctional Association.

Ostapuik, E. and Porteous, M.A. (1974) Psychiatric referrals in a regional assessment centre, Community Schools Gazette, 68, 264-275.

Rapoport, R. (1960) The Community as Doctor. London, Tavistock Publications.

Robison, J. and Smith, G. (1971) The effectiveness of correctional programs, Crime and Delinquency, 17, 67-80.

Scott, P.D. (1964) Approved School success rates, Brit. J. Criminol. 4, 525-556.

Sinclair, I.A.C. (1971) Hostels for Probationers. London, H.M.S.O.

Sinclair, I.A.C. and Clarke, R.V.G. (1973) Acting-out behaviour and its significance for the residential treatment of delinquents, J. Child Psychol. Psychiat. 14, 283-291.

Tutt, N. (1976) Recommittals of juvenile delinquents, Brit. J. Criminol. 16, 385-388.

Weeks, S. Ashley, (1958) Youthful Offenders at Highfields. Ann Arbor, University of Michigan Press.

Wills, W.D. (1971) Spare the Child: The Story of an Experimental Approved School. London, Penguin.

Wilson, H. (1975) Delinquents and non-delinquents in the inner city, Soc. Work Today, 5, 446-449.

AUTHOR INDEX

SUBJECT INDEX

Absconding 149, 150-151, 155
Achievement Place project
  127-131
Acting-out behaviour 145
Adolescents, EEGs in 13
Aggression
  and epilepy 17-20
  EEG abnormalities related
    to x
  "justified" 68-71
  measures of 79-82
  parental influence on
    children's 73-74
  persistent x
  provocation of ix
Ameliorating factors in conduct disorders 107
Antagonism between siblings
  55
Antisemitism 8-9
Approved schools 149, 150
  level of absconding from
  155
Assertive behaviour 117-118

Baby-battering 5
Barakumin peoples 4
Behaviour
  acting-out 145
  assertive 117-118
  at home 43-44
  at school 43
  characteristics 37, 39
  delinquent, causes of 152-
  153
  impact of institutional
    environment on 150
  modification 127, 153, 154
  reinforcement 118-119, 121,

122
  social 42
Behavioural
  change, maintenance of 133
  learning xi
  questionnaires 96
  treatment of conduct disorders
    115-135
Berkeley Guidance Study 74
Bossiness 55
Brain damage, organic 14
Bullying 33

Cambridge Study in Delinquent
  Development x, xi, 75
Causes of delinquent behaviour
  152-153
Child-battering 5
Childhood experience 5, 6, 9
Children in care 97-98
Children and Young Persons Act
  (1969) 143
Choice of treatments 153
CNS, delayed maturation of 2
Communalism 145
Community homes 143-156
  level of absconding from 155
Compensating circumstances 107
Concentration camps, cruelty
  and humiliation in 5
Conflict
  between parents and children
  129
  marital 89-90
Contingency contracting 144
Criminality of parents of delin-
  quents 77
Criminals, characteristics of
  152

167